*Empathy
and the Practice
of Medicine*

Empathy and the Practice of Medicine

BEYOND PILLS AND THE SCALPEL

EDITED BY
HOWARD M. SPIRO
MARY G. MCCREA CURNEN
ENID PESCHEL
DEBORAH ST. JAMES

Prepared under the auspices of
The Program for Humanities in Medicine
Yale University School of Medicine

Yale University Press
New Haven and London

Chapter 2 taken from *Annals of Internal Medicine* 116(1992):843–46. Used here with permission.

Set in Janson Text type by The Composing Room of Michigan, Inc. Printed in the United States of America by Vail-Ballou Press, Binghamton, New York.

Library of Congress Cataloging-in-Publication Data

Empathy and the practice of medicine : beyond pills and the scalpel /
edited by Howard M. Spiro . . . [et al.].
  p.   cm.
Includes bibliographical references and index.
ISBN 0-300-05840-3
  1. Physician and patient. 2. Medical personnel and patient.
3. Empathy. I. Spiro, Howard M. (Howard Marget), 1924– .
R727.3.R48 1993
610.69'6—dc20   93-27733
                                                  CIP

A catalogue record for this book is available from the British Library.
The paper in this book meets the guidelines for permanence and durability of the Committee on Production Guidelines for Book Longevity of the Council on Library Resources.

10   9   8   7   6   5   4   3   2   1

The illustration on the jacket is part of *A Three-Bed Hospital*, a fifteenth-century miniature from an illuminated manuscript in Ferrara. At the upper right, an attendant brings a bowl to a slightly doubtful patient; below, a physician cleanses an ugly-looking leg wound for an anxious outpatient. More than lance and potion, caring for the sick requires empathy and understanding (Florence, Biblioteca Medicea-Laurenziana, Gaddian MS 24, folio 247v. Avicenna, *Canon*, beginning of book IV).

One of the most tragic events of our time is that we know more than ever before the pains and sufferings of the world, and yet are less and less able to respond to them.

—Henri J. M. Nouwen

Contents

Foreword

If it can be said about any book that it is necessary, then *Empathy and the Practice of Medicine* is such a book. Technology has turned us into a race of medical pioneers, willing or not. So many crossroads; so many dilemmas. Using the soft words of husbandry—harvest and transplantation—our organs are donated and received from one to another, from species to species even. Fetal tissue is needled directly into the brain; fertilization is made to occur in a petri dish as a woman's egg is sprinkled with sperm. Is the sprinkler still to be regarded as the mate or the consort? Or shall he be called the depositor? An unromantic view of fatherhood, it would seem. We have not anticipated the avalanche of machinery and the data these machines produce, and so we have been left unprepared to make hard choices for ourselves and for our next-of-kin. *Empathy and the Practice of Medicine* can help us regain our footing.

The word *empathy* means the power of projecting one's personality into the object of contemplation, and so fully understanding it. Thus empathy is very different from sympathy or tenderness. The distinguished authors who have contributed to this book all place the responsibility and the privilege of awakening compassion for the sick directly upon those who do the tending—nurses and doctors. The book also explores technology's effect on ethics and questions whether the education and the desire to be empathic will hobble a physician's scientific objectivity: is it dangerous for a patient when a doctor becomes too empathic? Several of the authors show how the reading of literature can help doctors and nurses to become more empathic. Others tell stories to illustrate such a thesis. All in all, this is a brilliant and useful collection placed in the service of the patient and those who take care of the sick.

Acknowledgments

A remarkable group of distinguished medical writers have contributed generously to this book on empathy. The editors, from the Program for Humanities in Medicine at Yale University, thank each and all for sharing with us their thoughts, experiences, and suggestions on the important topic of the patient-doctor relationship.

We greatly appreciate the efficient and timely directorial assistance of Marla Benedetti and Tamma McNeill. Without their dedicated work, this book might not have seen the light of day.

To Dr. Edwin C. Cadman, chairman of the department of internal medicine at Yale Medical School, we express our gratitude for encouraging more empathy among faculty members, residents, students, and physicians in practice.

We are much indebted to Clara Gyorgyey and Priscilla W. Norton for the success of the Humanities in Medicine Lecture Series, which attracts an increasing number of members from the Medical School, other university departments, and the public at large. We are also grateful to Ferenc Gyorgyey, historical librarian, and Grethe Shepherd, from the Yale Medical Library, for suggesting the illustration for the cover.

Our thanks also goes to Jean Thomson Black, science editor at Yale University Press, and to her colleagues at the press who helped us in so many ways.

Last but not least, our gratitude goes to Miles, Inc., for supporting the publication of this book and distributing it to so many physicians in the United States.

*Empathy
and the Practice
of Medicine*

Chapter 1
Empathy: An Introduction

HOWARD M. SPIRO

A Case

A thirty-four-year-old woman from El Salvador who spoke little English and was severely deaf, had persistent abdominal pain and trouble swallowing. At the Primary Care Clinic she had been subjected to a computed tomography (CT) scan, ultrasound, and barium X-rays. She had seen the gynecologist, the otolaryngologist, the psychiatrist, and now the gastroenterologist. Through the translator it came out that her husband drank and had no job and that the one child she had had after three pregnancies suffered from spina bifida and was confined to a wheel chair and burdened with a urinary bag. The gastroenterologist, when asked whether bacteria in her stomach could account for her pains, wondered whether her physician felt that every pain had to have a site somewhere in the body.

This collection is the outgrowth of a talk I gave to the Yale Medical School Council, "What Is Empathy and Can It Be Taught?" Like any good academic, I desired to find some permanence for my words in print, so I sent the manuscript to a respected journal where the editor rejected it for reasons described in this volume (Landau). Its publication elsewhere (reprinted here as Chapter 2) brought enthusiastic letters from physicians that made clear how eager they

1

were to express their fellow-feelings for their patients, and how tired they were of detachment and equanimity. Hurt at the contempt heaped on them by critics of the medical care system and some of the public, they described how they still found joy in their work as doctors and how delighted they were that a university clinician would so praise empathy. Shortly afterwards, when the opportunity came for me, together with my colleagues in Yale's Program for Humanities in Medicine, to collect the chapters for this book, I took it as a chance to celebrate empathy—as a balance to equanimity.

The authors of the chapters in this volume are mainly physicians; a nurse and more than one Ph.D. have widened our view. All but one offer praise for empathy. The book has three sections: (1) empathy in practice, (2) empathy in teaching, and (3) empathy in theory. Yet in locating empathy in the physician, we may have ignored the patient, paradoxically enough. My psychiatrist daughter, Carolyn Spiro-Winn, asks, "How much does empathy begin in the patient?" The stories in the first section of this book may suggest the answer, once the question is posed.

I hope that this volume will enhance recognition of all the emotions in the practice of medicine, not empathy alone. Physicians can still be active healing agents: *disease*, which is what diagnostic equipment displays, needs science for cure, whereas *illness*, the patient's suffering, needs the physician for care.

Empathy and Equanimity

Empathy must joust with equanimity now that physicians are being turned into clerks and mechanics by a bureaucracy that regards "health care workers" as interchangeable modules. Financial constraints, of which "managed competition" is the latest example, look to measure out medical practice in units that can be weighed, delivered, and paid for like parcels. What cannot be so packaged counts for little. Empathy is the feeling that "I might be you" or "I am you," but it is more than just an intellectual identification; empathy must be accompanied by feeling. Sympathy brings compassion, "I want to help you," but empathy brings emotion. Without feeling there is no empathy.

In this book we praise empathy. Some have considered such praise a criticism of science, but that is a mistake. Medical practice is not an either-or situation. There are no dichotomies: clinicians need science *and* emotion, reason *and* intuition, technology *and* narratives, equanimity *and* empathy.

The Distrust of Empathy Today

TECHNOLOGY The power of technology and science has reduced the role of personal virtue or character in medical practice. Our technological triumphs have made many doctors feel so much like mere conduits of power that they no longer think of themselves as healing agents: pills are the gift of modern pharmaceutical research, diagnostic studies are carried out by remote computerized machinery like magnetic resonance imaging (MRI) that physicians only dimly understand, and what can now be done with wires and catheters dazzles the mind. CT scans and MRIS give us spectacular new views of the world, more beguiling than those from the moon. But modern cross-sectional images, like X-rays before them, can be turned into icons, giving precision at the cost of intimacy. To order a CT scan is easier—and far quicker—than listening to the patient, and more likely to deliver a picture of the disease, or at least of something inside the patient.

"TEAM" MEDICINE The impersonality of "team" medicine diffuses personal responsibility along with empathy in the hospital, and group practice weakens these qualities even in doctors' offices. Hospital practice has become so precise that many think it a waste of time, destructive even, for doctors to get emotionally involved with their patients. The algorithms of hospital care are stark and resolute; to feel emotion for patients would only get in the way of the tasks where only knowledge counts. In the past, doctors were merely observers in the night, but now they are truly warriors against death, and in hospital intensive care units (really intensive *cure* units) they never cease their battles. The corridors of Hope empty beside those of Action. Doctors and nurses are so busy in the hospital that there is no time for contemplation, only for delight in the correct diagnosis predicted, the mystery solved, death delayed. Empathy would only get in the way.

AUTONOMY The patient-autonomy movement in the 1960s brought the conviction that patients were equal partners with physicians in making medical decisions about themselves. Once the "captain of the ship," the doctor would order his patient (I use the masculine pronoun deliberately) to do as he directed until "informed consent" outmoded the paternalism that motivated physicians to assume responsibility. Even though parentalism, paternalism reborn, has lately been regaining some luster, doctors remain self-conscious about taking over and keep their distance.

MEDICAL TRAINING For many modern physicians, equanimity remains the model, as a virtue praised by Sir William Osler. Empathy gets drained out of medical students early in their academic careers. They get chosen for their victories, their grades, for scientific experience and energy. "Introspective" and "loving" are not adjectives that earn ready acceptance to most medical schools; the poets or writers who emerge use their medical training mainly for background. Training in molecular biology gives students only a microscopic and mechanical view of humankind. Yet even before molecular biology did so much to transform medical practice, physicians had already learned, "Don't get too involved. If you do, a little bit of you will die with each patient."

How can anyone who is not a surgeon still believe that a lone physician can be an active diagnostic or therapeutic agent? To suggest that the character of a doctor counts for much is to go against what happens in the hospitals. The trouble is, what is needed in hospitals is not what works in an office, and that is where alternative medicine has lessons for medical practice.

How to Strengthen Empathy

Where does empathy begin? Is it a quality of the physician only? Or does it reside in the patient? Can it be learned or is it innate? Is it only "counter-transference," as psychiatrists might aver? Is empathy possible for everyone, are everyone's receptors ready but "down-regulated," to use modern parlance, or must the right neural connections be formed early in life when the brain is still plastic? Are some doctors naturally *non*-empathic? Are some patients more "empathogenic" than others? Are there truly hateful patients—or physicians—who cannot love, whom no one can love? Should medical students choose their careers on the basis of their character as much as their skills? Do time and age bring empathy along with serenity? Does experience count in truly caring for the sick, or does it fade away with habit?

THE EAR: LISTENING TO THE PATIENT'S STORY   Social medicine and psychosomatic medicine, so full of promise in the 1940s, faded with the triumphs of science and molecular biology. It is hard to remember how little doctors could do to treat patients in the 1940s, yet patient-doctor relationships have changed little in the last fifty years. As studies repeatedly show, most people still go to physicians looking for help for existential pains, for the suffering of living in this world, for ailments that no technology can correct. That is where the patient's story comes in, for it can reveal what is important in the images the doctor obtains. The physician's first and most important task is to decide what is going on, what tests must be done, if any. At the same time, doctors must listen to what the patient tells them, remaining open to be moved by the story even, for that will often clear the path to diagnosis. Listening goes straight to the heart and helps to create empathy. Empathy opens our eyes to let us see what the CT scan has missed. The ear is as important as the eye in medical practice. Is it too much to claim that the physician must be the mediator between the images and the patient?

SICK DOCTORS When physicians fall sick they learn the value of empathy (Mandell and Spiro 1987); they discover how great a price they have paid for suppressing emotions: most of us no longer know when we have feelings. Imperturbability long practiced brings "alexithymia," a failure to recognize feelings when you have them. Most sick doctors ignore their problems, deny their very real disability, and then come to lament their isolation from their imperturbable colleagues. Moreover, physicians still healthy are glad not to confront the sickness of a colleague, for it signals their own mortality. One reason why "No Visitors" signs appear so automatically when doctors are admitted to the hospital may be to permit their colleagues to pass by without feeling guilt, the one emotion doctors still allow.

PATHOGRAPHY The chapters in this book suggest how empathy can be retained and strengthened through reading, through studying the humanities, and through conversation. Just as artists learn to see by drawing, so doctors can learn empathy by putting themselves in their patients' place. That does not mean suffering through tubes or tests; it means trying to feel the story as the patient feels it. "Pathography," the stories of illness from the inside, help nourish empathy. When medical students and physicians write accounts of the way they imagine patients live their "case histories," they may begin to feel what the patients feel. When they read accounts of what it is like to be sick, empathy can grow—but only if discussion follows reading. That is where the study of humanities comes in: to read great works of fiction is to widen experience readily, to find our patients in the stories of the masters. Yet there is so little time in the curriculum for more than science. Later, in practice, there is far more emphasis on doing than on contemplating, so that, sadly enough, wide reading is not part of the physician's life. Anthropology and sociology, which might help physicians understand how culture affects the interpretation of pain, are not encouraged in graduate courses. The busy clinician orders a CT scan for the patient whose language he or she cannot speak and requests a consultation.

CONVERSATION Talking is crucial. Empathy withers in silence. Talking about feelings helps students and residents find where they have hidden empathy during training. Talking makes empathy plausible, even respectable, if we are too embarrassed to admit the feelings that lie just below our equanimity. At an ethics conference in a small community hospital not too long ago, a resident burst out, "I envy people who believe in God," and that cry has not been forgotten by those who heard him. Conversation strengthens empathy. In the end, empathy is a two-way street, a wrestling that Buber called the "I and Thou," and it is needed as much today as ever before.

References

Mandell, H., and H. Spiro. 1987. *When Doctors Get Sick*. New York: Plenum.

Osler, W. 1932. *Aequanimitas with Other Addresses to Medical Students, Nurses, and Practitioners of Medicine*. 3d ed. Philadelphia: Blakiston.

Stoeckle, J. D., I. K. Zola, and G. E. Davidson. 1964. The quantity and significance of psychological distress in medical patients. *Journal of Chronic Disease*. 17:959–70.

Chapter 2
What Is Empathy and
Can It Be Taught?

HOWARD M. SPIRO

A medical student told how he and a group of residents were laughing and joking through "work-rounds" one morning; they expressed amused resentment toward their next patient, a comatose old man awaiting his PEG (percutaneous endoscopic gastrostomy) ticket to a "nursing warehouse." After the ritual chest examination and a few shouts in his ear, they turned to go, when their attention was caught by a new card on the wall, colored by a child's hand. "Get well soon, Grandpa," it read. The troupe fell silent as they left the room, and for a moment the joking ceased. That was empathy, with the child if not with the old man.

Empathy is the feeling that persons or objects arouse in us as projections of our feelings and thoughts. It is evident when "I and you" becomes "I am you," or at least "I might be you." Empathy has fascinated philosophers and art critics, psychiatrists and psychologists (Book 1988), but modern physicians have shown less interest in this "almost magical" phenomenon (C. S. Spiro, unpublished) and have instead preferred equanimity. Empathy, however, underlies the qualities of the humanistic physician and should frame the skills of all professionals who care for patients.

7

Definitions

Empathy has two faces, the esthetic and the personal (Gauss 1973). As medicine becomes more visual, the esthetic aspect has lessons for physicians. Empathy is what we feel when we see a picture that moves us. However, to recognize a baseball in a picture, or sadness in a face, one must have held a ball or felt sad. Guides to empathy come from the arts, where the concept was first elaborated (Gauss 1973). A "method" actor is "transfigured" by his or her part so that, as someone put it, the audience sits entranced by the illusion. The stage-hands behind the scene, however, find no illusions, only a job. Medical school squeezes empathy out of our students as we take them "backstage" in the body.

Empathy is, however, much more than illusion. Empathy is more than know-ing what we see; it is the emotion generated by the image. It is difficult to distinguish empathy from sympathy: where empathy feels "I am you" sympathy may well mean "I want to help you." Sympathy involves compassion but not passion. As a medical student has suggested, empathy means "I *could be* you." John Donne knew empathy when he admonished, the "bell tolls for thee." Others in the religious tradition, like Martin Buber when he explored the "I and thou," also guide us to it.

For Freud, empathy was the "mechanism by means of which we are enabled to take up any attitude at all towards another mental life" (Freud 1955, 110). For Jung, projection accounts for empathy and includes a merging of the viewer with the viewed. Harries has called empathy "a feeling of being at home with the object contemplated," as a friend and not as a stranger (K. Harries quoted in Hogenson 1981, 69).

Empathy requires living and knowing. Those who see empathy as a neuro-biologic response (Brothers 1989) that depends on learned experience will point to the way in which we are compelled to imitate someone who yawns or to the way in which the smell of vomit evokes nausea. Those biologic responses, sympathetic as they may be, do not define empathy, but they do yield clues. Empathy must be more than identification, because empathy brings with it feeling. The purge of emotions that Aristotle in his *Poetics* called catharsis depends on empathy (Aristotle 1938).

Losing Empathy in Training: Expertise

Empathy helps us to know who we are and what we feel. Nowhere is the old saw, "if you don't use it, you lose it," truer. During medical education, we first teach the students science, and then we teach them detachment. To these barriers to human understanding, they later add the armor of pride and the fortress of a desk between themselves and their patients. As I know them, college students start out with much empathy and genuine love—a real desire to help other people. In medical school, however, they learn to mask their feelings, or worse, to deny them. They learn detachment and equanimity. The increased emphasis on molecular biology to the exclusion of the humanities encourages students to focus not on patients, but on diseases. A desk, Nagel reminds us, is more than its spaces and electrons (Nagel 1961).

In the twenty-first century, as technology triumphs, empathy will need more attention than equanimity. Maybe the world of medicine always lay apart from the world of others, but science was once a puny force that had little attraction for those wishing to care for the sick. In the twentieth century, however, much has been learned. The advances in science have been so transfixing and the acceleration of knowledge has grown so compelling that Nagel's desk has lost its solidity. Physicians need to relearn the body, and empathy can help us to regain our feeling.

The role and character of the patient have remained virtually unchanged; however, what we physicians can do to patients is vastly more effective than before. Although history taking differs little from fifty years ago, the modes of treatment have changed radically. (If I treated patients the way I was taught back then, the lawyers would soon be at my door.) In medical school, the primary world of science beguiles us with new ways of looking at the body, new languages, and new technologies. Medical students put on new costumes to differentiate themselves from the world of those outside the profession. Other professionals are changed as much, but few expect much empathy from lawyers or accountants.

Students begin their medical education with a cargo of empathy, but we teach them to see themselves as experts, to fix what is damaged, and to "rule out" disease in their field. The phrase, "I dress the wound, God heals it," was once used to proclaim confidence in the Creator, but it now more aptly describes the focus of the specialist: "I do what I am trained to do."

Medical students begin their education with the dead body and the living cell; they learn that the patient is passive and that the cells are alive. Dissection of a cadaver in medical school teaches primacy of the eye over the ear, for cadavers do not complain, and no one has to listen. It is then that students first learn to harden themselves against empathy.

Empathy overcomes narcissism and isolation. We physicians are trained in narcissism, but we have to know who we are to find ourselves and to confirm ourselves in others. Modern medicine has turned physicians away from themselves and toward the contemplation of images. These images include only the body and its various systems and structures and do not show the mind and spirit of the patient.

Conversation helps to develop empathy, for it is here that we learn of shared experiences and feelings; "in empathy one discovers oneself in the object of contemplation" (Hogenson 1981, 69). Medical students, however, have little time to discover and to enlarge themselves, and residents are fatigued on the wards. Despite their immersion in molecular biology or technology, students and residents will someday care for patients who are not generalizable in the ways of science. Yet, the training of doctors today sometimes seems akin to the training of would-be tailors in the chemistry of cotton and wool, in the methods of shearing, and in the linkage of polyester chains. When future tailors ask about the cutting of patterns, they might be told, "When you learn how cloth is made, you'll know how to make a suit."

We doctors are selected by victories: We reached college because we were bright and competitive in high school, and we reached medical school through competition and hard-edged achievements. We are taught that hard work brings all the answers—and all the rewards. Residencies teach the same tough message. Residency training quenches the embers of empathy. Isolation, long hours of service, chronic lack of sleep, sadness at prolonged human tragedies, and depression at futile and often incomprehensible therapeutic maneuvers turn even the most empathic of our children from caring physicians into tired terminators. No wonder we have little empathy for the defeated, the humble, the dying, those who have not made it to the top of the heap, and even for the sick. Our energy gets us into medical school and after that little time remains for contemplation.

Even for the medical faculty, occasions for spontaneous collegiality have diminished under the pressure of research grants or diagnostic machinery. My medical school has no faculty club, nor even a doctors' dining room, a place where physicians and teachers can exchange ideas at leisure. Elegant centers exist for study and an ever increasing number of laboratories are provided for molecular research, but these are structures only for scientific collaboration and cooperation. Meeting our colleagues in an unstructured way, as people, has become much more difficult. Work is everything, so little time remains for contemplation, and none remains for the humanities.

In clinical medicine, we talk mostly about the "case" and not about the person; reports are written in the passive voice to imply that truth is being uncovered by an ineluctable force. The style of medical writing is "objective" and impersonal, where that which can be seen is given more importance than what can be heard. The eye is quicker than the ear; yet, the patient's experience is more complicated and variable than the disease visible to the doctor. Often the individual patient is seen as only a model, a body to be treated, or a good "teaching case" that illustrates a point.

Artists discover themselves in their work (Berger 1971); they uncover the subject in their drawing or painting. In the same way, taking a case history can be a discovery for the physician. As abstraction in art represents withdrawal, however, the abstraction of disease may distance us from the patient. I find little ecstasy in a cubist painting, and it is difficult to feel empathy for the computed tomographic image of a stranger with pancreatic cancer. "Great case!" we are likely to exclaim as we look for the dilated common duct.

Restoring Empathy

Can empathy be taught? Is it a gift or a skill? Is it verbal or visual? How can we express it? How can we make ourselves more empathic? A better question might be, "Can we recover the empathy we once had?" The brain may establish most of its connections during childhood, but recent evidence has shown that new connections can form late in life, although more slowly. Medical students and physicians may yet be able to retain and enhance their natural empathy. That goal, however, requires the consideration of human life and experience; the reading of stories and novels; and the discussion of narratives, paintings, and even role models (Hunter 1986; Hawkins 1992). It also requires more collegiality with our students and resident physicians as much as with each other. If we abuse our residents with too much work, they will learn to care less for their patients, and too much for themselves.

Empathy can be strengthened best through stories. In his farewell speech at Yale Medical School, Chaplain Bill Coffin told how, when he was sick and miserable with pneumonia, he shrank away from the radiance of the jolly, confident physicians standing over him. They were too healthy for him. That story has changed the way in which I deal with the sick.

Medical students have not yet, even in these times, had all possible experiences. Baudelaire said, "Every experience is a good experience," but we hope that our children will be spared a few. If empathy depends on experience, then that is the area in which novels, fiction, stories, and paintings can enlarge empathy. Clinical tales, as Oliver Sacks calls them, are the most important; to look at a painting is, however, sometimes to be fooled.

The humanities surely need no justification on a utilitarian basis: the colleges are more important to our land than are the medical schools. The utilitarian calculus of medical school, however, demands a "cost-benefit" analysis, because the medical faculty have forgotten Aristotle's admonition, to know when it is wiser not to measure something.

It would be presumptuous to add to what has already been written about medical school and graduate training. Talk about the curriculum, like philosophy, aims too much at some standard student with little passion and less identity. Rhetoric, the old art of persuasion, needs a rebirth in medical practice (Spiro 1986). Physicians are more than conduits of pills or procedures, and they should be more than transparent technicians; to quote the old phrase, they need character.

Emphasis on History Taking Can Enhance Empathy

History taking is more than one person interviewing another: Histories are taken, and they are received. Doctors shape stories using constraints of form or purpose, and histories are transmitted in many ways (Donnelly 1986). The age of the patient or of the physician, the purpose of the history, the interest or specialty of the physician, whether the history is the first or the fifth one taken, what we allow ourselves to feel, and what we have become, are all important determinants of the written record. Of course, physicians vary in their skills and gifts. Some are better at hand-eye coordination and others, at visual perception; some are born with empathy and others, the "alexithymic," cannot feel their own emotions or may not have any. Medical students bring different skills to the profession; some prove to be poor surgeons, whereas others lack the interpersonal skills upon which to build clinical expertise. Would-be physicians should become as aware of these matters as they are of the enzyme systems of the liver. The ways in which differing cultures regard disease are equally important, although they may be the stuff of popular culture (Payer 1988). (The *Lancet* has recently devoted a new section to medical anthropology.) Body language is no less important. The clues that make the physician aware at the first meeting that a patient is depressed require free-floating attention, as psychoanalysts call it, but such a skill must be cultivated. Students should think about their metaphors for a physician: Is a doctor a scientist, a detective, a parent, or just an expert called in to be a "fixer"?

The relocation of residency training from the hospitals back to the outpatient clinics where it began (to the clinics of the poor where it could be found 100 years ago) will not in itself strengthen empathy. Training in continuing care will be of little value without doctors who know something of the life of the people whom they serve; who can empathize with immigrants from Asia and Mexico, with the Southern or ghetto experience; and who know of the Holocaust and of communist oppression.

Many physicians of my generation, trained to worship the icons of X-ray films, find it difficult to accept that abdominal pain may come from life as well as from the liver. Yet, in the world of literature (outside our medical schools with their emphasis on objectivity) a new genus of "pathography," the story of persons with disease, has sounded an antiphony that may help (Hunter 1986; Hawkins 1992). The anecdotes of pathography tell the narrative of what patients feel and suffer in their bodies. When the origin of pain puzzles us—and even when it does not—it may be helpful to ask the patient what he or she thinks is wrong. Yet, a respected clinical scientist recently asked, "How often does the patient really know the diagnosis?" He had lost the point, that patients usually know the circumstances of their illness, at least at first, in greater detail than does the physician. Science looks toward the general, but physicians deal with the particular. The individual is lost among our statistics and archetypes. Hunter (1986) has pointed out that the physician begins by getting a story from a patient but that the physician then "abstracts" the patient or, as Baron (1981) has put it, the patient is subtracted and becomes transparent. The patient is put in parentheses.

Thomas (1974) has justly claimed that it is cheaper to find the cause of a disease than to pay for various intermediate forms of care. Thomas was, however, a pathologist, and for pathologists the eye counts for more than the ear. The problems of living—existential, socioeconomic, and emotional—that account for 80 percent of visits to physicians' offices represent complaints that are unlikely to be switched on or off by an aberrant gene.

I do not propose to pile stories of illness or pathographies atop the already overloaded curriculum. Discussed by sympathetic faculty as fervently as the latest report from the "literature," such stories would teach students what it is to be a patient and what it is to be a doctor (Hawkins 1992). First- and second-year students are eager for such bridges between our two worlds. By their third or fourth year, however, they have little time and less enthusiasm for anecdotes, because by this time they have taken on our "medical" values.

We cannot have all the experiences possible; however, to take a current example, John Updike (1990) can teach us much about what it is like to have a heart attack or to be a lover with psoriasis. Reading, of course, must be accompanied by conversations that broaden the vistas available to us if we listen.

Conversation may be the key. Continuing discussions about patient-doctor relationships and about human relationships in general throughout medical school (especially in the final two skill-sharpening years) and during residency will fan the passion of empathy. No lectures, please; case discussions about our patients, their stories, and about ourselves will help more than dry-as-dust doctrine.

Restoring Passion

Should equanimity be so widely praised for all physicians? Detachment has been much lauded since Osler, but is it as helpful to the internist as to the surgeon? Whom does it help? Too much emotion in medical practice can be destructive; passion needs control. However, these matters need discussion as much as do somatostatin receptors. My generation, for example, learned little about the sexual habits of those other than our partners; as medical students we were taught not to intrude with questions about sex, surprising as that might now seem. In the 1960s, we learned to ask more intimate questions, and, although we found it difficult at first, we later learned how easy and helpful such inquiry proved. Now, we must restore to medicine the passion that has been forced out by equanimity.

Doctors prefer dichotomies: right or left, up or down, physician or patient, you or I. Medicine is, however, both science and narrative, both reason and intuition. Empathy may yet prove essential in the third millennium, when we have relegated computers to routine diagnosis. Computed tomographic scans offer no compassion, and magnetic resonance imaging has no human face. Only men and women are capable of empathy.

References

Aristotle. 1938. *Poetics*, ed. W. D. Ross. New York: Scribners.

Baron, R. J. 1981. Bridging clinical distance: An empathic rediscovery of the known. *Journal of Medical Philosophy*. 6:5–23.

Berger, J. 1971. Drawing. In *The Look of Things*. New York: Viking Press.

Book, H. E. 1988. Empathy: Misconceptions and misuses in psychotherapy. *American Journal of Psychiatry*. 145:420–24.

Brothers, L. 1989. A biological perspective on empathy. *American Journal of Psychiatry*. 146:10–19.

Donnelly, W. J. 1986. Righting the medical records: Transforming chronicle into story. *Journal of the American Medical Association*. 260:823–25.

Freud, S. 1955. Group psychology and the analysis of the ego. In *The Standard Edition of the Complete Psychological Works of Sigmund Freud*, ed. and trans. J. Strachey, vol. 18. London: Hogarth Press.

Gauss, C. E. 1973. Empathy. In *Dictionary of the History of Ideas*, ed. P. Wiener. New York: Scribners. 2:85–89.

Hawkins, A. H. 1992. Restoring the patient's voice: The case of Gilda Radner. *Yale Journal of Biology and Medicine*. 65:173–81.

Hogenson, G. B. 1981. Depth psychology, death and the hermeneutic of empathy. *Journal of Medical Philosophy*. 6:67–89.

Hunter, K. M. 1986. "There was this one guy . . .": The uses of anecdotes in medicine. *Perspectives in Biology and Medicine*. 29:619–30.

Nagel, E. 1961. *The Structure of Science: Problems in the Logic of Scientific Explanation*. New York: Harcourt Brace & World.

Payer, L. 1988. *Medicine and Culture*. New York: Holt.

Spiro, H. M. 1986. *Doctors, Patients, and Placebos*. New Haven: Yale University Press.

Thomas, L. 1974. The technology of medicine. In *The Lives of a Cell*. New York: Bantam Books.

Updike, J. 1990. *Rabbit at Rest*. New York: Knopf.

Part One
The Practice of
Empathy

These first stories plunge the reader into the physician's daily maelstrom: people age, lose their powers, die too often and too slowly; children are maimed in spirit and body, crippled by absent parents and wretched cities; not everyone wins the race. Doctors, who see only those who have fallen behind, take these events as the workings of a malign Fate: hardworking men and women in our tough times lose their jobs and their houses and wonder what has happened; alcohol and drugs destroy so many for reasons so unsure while the doctors watch, patching here and there.

Later, the anguish fades as experiences repeated over and over drain away empathy. Empathy is so easy to lose; to study the liver enzymes many years ago, I had to kill rats without using any anesthesia, cracking their heads against the side of the table. In order to kill the rats, I learned to hate them. Doctors do not learn hate, but they do learn to lose their feelings; guilt is the only emotion that physicians allow themselves to enjoy.

The authors in this first section show that loss of empathy is not inevitable. George S. Bascom sketches stories from his life as a small-town surgeon with humor as well as with compassion. His has been a life well spent, friend as well as surgeon to his patients, citizen as well as physician, finding stories on "both sides of the examining room door."

In his tribute to a close friend, a physician with a chest tumor, John Stone shows the identification that goes with empathy. More than that, his essay shows how doctors do not have to wall off their emotions, but then Stone is a poet as well as a doctor.

I wept, truly, when I first read the "real stories" that Joanne Lynn tells of her work in nursing homes and in hospices with people who are dying or disabled. These tales of the aged, of those who suffer, of people—not patients—dying of cancer or AIDS, have as much to teach physicians as anything in more formal literature. Sadness pervades Lynn's accounts; but jubilation is also present. "It is an extraordinary privilege to have been allowed to travel in the valley of death with about two thousand patients." She has learned the lessons of death and is not embarrassed to talk about it.

Finally, like C. S. Lewis in the *Screwtape Letters*, Michael LaCombe has "found" a new letter from a devil advising his student how to trap the soul of a doctor by using truth-telling and virtue as snares. To get physicians to put their own merit above their patients' comfort, his devil seeks to replace emotions with equanimity and objectivity; as physicians slide from enjoying their work to being proud of what they are, they begin to mistake the disease for the patient and are lost. As LaCombe puts it, doctors "cannot feel, and more important they scorn feeling." For the devil, empathy is the enemy, for it reminds physicians who will listen of what Wordsworth called the "still, sad music of humanity."

H. M. S.

Chapter 3
Sketches from a
Surgeon's Notebook

GEORGE S. BASCOM

When I came home to practice, the first patient I saw was Orville Burtis. He was a weathered cattleman and an old family friend who had chosen a complete physical exam as a way of welcoming me. I occupied a pair of rooms on the second floor of a fine old pressed-brick home. Below was a busy waiting room and the offices of my father and Willard Schwartz and John Fairchild. They were primary care physicians, G.P.'s. Each had a different slant. Willard was an internist of volatile mood, and John was a cigarette-smoking anesthetist of very few words. My father's particular interest was surgery and obstetrics. But each doctor offered general care to families. My father was good at what he did. He had a Ph.D. in anatomy and a lively intelligence, and he was devoted to his patients.

Ours was a small town where the distinction between patient and friend was blurred. This had its drawbacks. Orville's office appointment was his way of greeting me and expressing his confidence in my skills. I understood that and did not charge him for the service, though I think he finally insisted on paying me five dollars. Friendship can make negotiations like this complicated. I had noticed my father's faithful but privately exasperated responses to hypochondriacal friends. It was unthinkable he should be haughty or cavalier. He accepted the fact that he was stuck with them.

But it had advantages, too. People understood his need for rest and leisure. They were generous and considerate in turn. So the practice atmosphere I grew up with and expected to enjoy and sometimes suffer was one of friendship.

Certainly other styles are open to a surgeon. Some are autocratic, some prayerful, some patronizing, some overbearing, some punctilious, some exceedingly formal. Some styles are appropriate, some inappropriate, but many serve to minimize personal involvement. In managed health care systems, the surgeon may have only a brief operative and postoperative exposure to the patient. It is efficient. It saves time and emotion.

But allow me to mourn the loss to both the patient and the doctor. Let me mourn the dance of the anesthetized surgeon over the anesthetized patient. Remoteness reduces the patient to a problem and the surgeon to a robot. Both miss the reward that often follows the venture of illness in which both patient and doctor are vulnerable and both need understanding. The surgeon misses a rich and various symphony, the unheard music Orville Burtis brought to the examining room—remembered stories by fire and lamplight, potluck suppers at his ranch, the death of his boy Dave, shingling his barn on a perfect day. The stories are wonderful. Stories wait on both sides of the examining room door. Sure, there is a medical problem to be addressed. But there are other issues, too.

Trust

Joel was a college professor, a writer, and a dramatist. He had a duodenal ulcer with recurrent pain and trouble enough to justify a vagotomy and pyloroplasty. He had tried everything in the way of conservative management and now was ready to consider surgery. But he was uneasy. How competent was I? How safe and effective was the procedure? More than that, and unspoken—perhaps even unconscious—was the matter of trust in my goodwill. Could he put his life in the hands of a stranger? As a man of imagination, he must have wondered who lived behind the features of my face. I could feel the struggle going on in Joel. It took time and several talks during which he covered some of the same questions more than once. After weeks of deliberation and careful thought, he decided on surgery.

I was impressed with his courage. Recognition of his struggle laid a heavy responsibility on me. His question became my own: Was I to be trusted? It made me more careful when Joel went to sleep and lay under the drapes and operating room lights. That question surfaces again and again, especially in cases where indications are blurred or risks and benefits nearly balanced. Joel's struggle to trust led to a reciprocal effort to be worthy of it. I tried to catch that in the following poem:

Joel
Long jawed friend
Your sleep seemed sound
Beneath the bright swift blade
Gliding silently
Not like a kinky saw
In soggy wood
But gliding silently
Cleaving your flesh
Like a skimmer.
The scalpel was busy
With its revelations
Trustingly.
The questions, reflections
Inquiries, decisions
Consultations and advice
Came down to that.
And I who sliced
My index finger
Deeply once in surgery
Have learned that trust
Which goes more swift and deep
Than shiny blades
Can also cut
Both ways.

Layla was another lesson. She had had multiple Caesarean sections and a failed hernia repair in Baghdad. Now a graduate student at Kansas State, she wanted the recurrence repaired. But, as I came to learn, she was incapable of trust. Her first two preoperative visits were a year apart. I suspect she spent the intervening time nourishing dark suspicions to help them grow. Why she elected me as her surgeon I cannot fathom. Probably it was because of my brother's kindness and courtesy to international students. Charlie was a physician in student health at Kansas State.

The surgery was scheduled after I called two Iraqi physicians in distant places, San Diego and Dallas, at her insistence. She demanded they be fully informed and concur with the operation. One was a dermatologist and the other a plastic surgeon, so the reassurance they offered had less to do with their competence than with their national origin. It was annoying to make these calls, but I thought it reasonable in view of her alien status and our unfamiliar customs. I explained the indications, recited the plans, and received heavily accented approval from her consultants.

By the time Layla reached the operating room I had the strong presentiment a recurrence would result in formidable turmoil. As an extra precaution, I decided to use Marlex mesh. It lay beautifully beneath the peritoneum when I had finished placing a ring of mattress sutures around the defect. The abdominal wall closed over the mesh without tension, and I was very pleased with the procedure. But Layla did not do well. She began to vomit, became increasingly uncomfortable and increasingly suspicious that I had done something wrong. I assured her she was getting all the fluids she needed intravenously. I apologized for the nasogastric tube and tried to make it as comfortable as possible. But Layla's suspicion was like obsidian, hard and impenetrable.

"Call my doctors," was her sullen response to my attempts at reassurance.

So I made call after call to faraway cities—Washington, D.C., New Orleans, even London. Some of these Middle Eastern consultants were surprised to get my call and were cordially supportive of what we were doing. Others acted as if they had been briefed by Layla, muttering noncommittal responses that breathed the same deep doubt about my judgment.

Layla got worse. Finally there was no question she was totally obstructed and needed reexploration. I proposed it to her and explained with all the patience I could command. "Call my doctors," she said, handing me the names of two new ones.

"Mrs. A.," I said. "There is no doubt in my mind about this. We do not need more advice. You need the operation now. If you are not satisfied, I want to turn your case over to a surgeon in whom you have confidence."

She stared at me. She and her husband, a large, rough-looking man, said they would let me know. In a few minutes the nurse gave me the word that they agreed and wanted me to carry on. So Layla came back to surgery. When I opened her abdomen, I found bowel stuck up against the mesh. It was distended proximally, collapsed distally. We freed it, interposed omentum between the mesh and her viscera, and Layla made an uneventful recovery. I saw her at the usual intervals after surgery. Each visit was an ordeal of few words. Her unshaken conviction remained that I was both negligent and incompetent. Her ingratitude was uncompromising, her dissatisfaction unwavering. When she was dismissed, I felt a great weight lift from my soul. I wanted never to see Layla again. And if, as some suggest, our feelings are a mirror of the patient's, she was glad to be rid of me.

Absurdity

Absurdity is no stranger to the patient-doctor relationship. Occasionally, I was asked to make a house call on a sorority girl. I remember as a college boy being acutely aware of the inviolate barrier between the first floor of the sorority house and the rooms above. No man dared breach that line between the public activity of the young women and the private—and richly imagined—activity above. Enough of that feeling lingered that some effort was needed to act casual when I arrived with my black medical bag. I marched up the carpeted stairs accompanied by the housemother and one or two of the senior sorority girls. "Man on second," someone called. I tried not to blush. Heads poked out the doors along the corridor and a bevy of young women in curlers and pajamas gathered behind us as we proceeded to the room of the patient. A drama suddenly mushroomed. The young girl had gastroenteritis and a stomachache, but she threw herself into suffering. The slightest touch to her discreetly bared abdomen elicited a cry of anguish and a writhing withdrawal. Her sisters, appreciative of her histrionics, reciprocated with cries and moans of sympathy. Surrounded by nubile loveliness and emotionally inundated, I examined and questioned her with increasing embarrassment, an embarrassment heightened by their hanging so on every word. It became opéra bouffe. Yes, I should have cleared the room and taken charge. But I was young, and the part was new to me. I had never before been the man on second.

And there was the matter of informed consent. Kansas State University with its excellent agriculture and engineering departments attracts many international students. One cannot help feeling a lot of sympathy for them when they get sick or need surgery. Here they are, thousands of miles from home in an alien culture, often short of funds and having to fend for themselves in a strange tongue. So I take particular pains to be respectful and to answer questions.

The young Iranian graduate student in engineering was yellow as a pumpkin. A work-up revealed gallstones. The presumption was that one had slipped into the common duct, blocked it, and was now causing his jaundice. He was a clean-shaven, intelligent, handsome young man. The whites of his dark brown eyes were deep yellow.

I sensed his English was imperfect, so I resolved to take particular care to explain everything, not fearing a lawsuit for failure to inform but out of the nobler impulse of Christian charity. I confess to feeling rather good about myself as I sat down with him at the nurse's station.

"Your surgery is scheduled for tomorrow morning," I began. "As your surgeon it is my duty to answer all your questions and explain fully what you can expect. Do you understand?"

"Yeah, sure. Sure."

"O.K. Do you know what the gallbladder is?"

"Sure. Sure."

"Well, your gallbladder contains stones which have formed from elements of your bile. You understand?"

"Sure."

"The gallbladder is a side arm, a reservoir off the main bile duct. It stores bile between meals and thickens it like syrup on the stove." I noticed his brow wrinkle a bit and thought perhaps I was going a little too fast. "Do you understand what I mean?"

He nodded. "Yeah. Sure."

Feeling a little doubtful, I explained that a stone had slipped into the main bile duct and blocked it. "That is why your skin and your eyes have turned yellow. The bile is backed up in your system. It can empty adequately only through the common duct." I looked at him again. "You understand?"

"Sure, sure."

"Now," I said, taking a deep breath, "An infection has developed in your bile ducts. Do you know what I mean by infection? Do you know what bacteria are?" I wondered if I was being a bit condescending.

He nodded. Did he look faintly bored?

"Well, this infection will come back again and again until the stones are removed from your common bile duct. We plan to remove the gallbladder and also remove the stones from your main bile duct. That will relieve the yellow jaundice and prevent more infections. Okay?"

"Yeah. Okay."

"Now I am required to tell you about problems or complications that you might have. Surgery doesn't always turn out perfectly. Sometimes an infection will occur inside the abdomen or under the skin. It doesn't happen often, but it can make you stay in the hospital longer." He looked a little troubled. "If it does happen, we can take care of it. Okay?"

"Sure." He nodded again.

"Any time we operate we can have some unexpected bleeding. Not often, of course. But it can happen. I have never had this trouble with a gallbladder."

He continued to meet my eyes and nod.

"Now, I must inform you that you could even die as a result of the surgery." He seemed to look more intently. I hurried on. "It is very unlikely. Very unlikely. About as risky as driving to Topeka. You know, anytime you drive to Topeka you could have a fatal accident. Sometimes people are killed on the highway, but it is so unlikely we don't worry about it. That's about the risk of your surgery."

He continued to look at me intently. "Do you have any questions?" I asked.

"Yeah," he answered, "when I go Topeka?"

Anger

Like absurdity, anger can dominate the relationship. Years ago while making rounds I was called to the emergency room. It lay at the end of a long corridor leading from the surgical floor. Wild with anger, a man's voice came racketing down the hall as I walked toward it. "Let go of me you fucking bitches. Goddamn you, fucking sons of bitches, get away from me!" And on and on. In the background was the sound of voices trying to pacify him. I saw a tangle of bodies when I entered. He was a large, lean young man with a scalp laceration. Ambulance attendants, nurses, and a policeman were trying to keep him on his back. He was bucking and cursing, trying to fling them away. He spat at one of the nurses, and I felt fury rise in me.

"You lie still," I shouted at him.

"Fuck you, you son of a bitch," he screamed. I could smell the liquor on his breath.

A friend had shown me a judo hold that involved grasping the fingers of the hand and separating them forcefully. He assured me it would pacify anyone. He had applied it to me, and I agreed. It was very painful.

Infuriated, I grasped the fingers of his right hand and separated them hard. And with pleasure. I expected him to quiet down, but he writhed around on the table until his bloodshot eyes were inches from mine. "Go ahead," he shrieked, "break them, you fucking bastard."

Shocked by my own savagery, I dropped his hand and stepped away. I was ashamed, humiliated. I felt others in the emergency room looking at me. "You'll have to jail him," I told the policeman. "We can't treat him this way. Bring him back when he sobers up."

I walked away as his cursing and yelling continued. He may have come back. Maybe someone more skilled in managing a berserk drunk came along and sutured his cut. I was glad to get away from him and from myself.

On another occasion anger broke out. It was one or two in the morning, a hot summer night, and I was tired from busy days and nights, lots of surgery and heavy office schedules and, of course, the damned emergency room. Theoretically we took emergency call in turn. But some cheated. Others of us, perhaps self-righteously, took up the slack, felt abused and rather noble, and sincerely hoped the community and hospital staff would notice and give us our due in terms of respect and loyalty. That is, we hoped the other lazy bastards would pay in the end.

So when the phone rang, even before I picked up the receiver, I was groaning inwardly. "Dr. Bascom," I answered.

"This is Memorial E.R., Dr. Bascom. We have a twenty-four-year-old male with a black widow spider bite on the arm."

"A black widow?"

"That's what he says."

"All right," I agreed reluctantly. "I'll be up."

"Thank you, Dr. Bascom." I hear real relief in the nurse's voice. It occurs to me I may be the fourth or fifth one she has called. By then it is too late to ask, and I find it easier just to get up and go.

I walk into a brightly lit ER and find a young man in dirty work clothes lounging against the examining table in the center of the tiled room. "What's the problem?" I snap. In the car I had asked myself if a black widow spider bite is really a surgical disease. I began to suspect a few primary care physicians had turned it down.

"A black widow spider bite," says the young man already offended by my tone. He looks fine. I detect the odor of beer.

"Are you sure it was a black widow?"

"It was black and had a red dot on its belly."

Suddenly his companion speaks. He is an equally scruffy, unwashed type who has been fidgeting as he leaned against a stainless steel counter. "It was a bee," he declares, responding angrily to my unsympathetic manner.

"A bee," I explode. "Well, what is it? A spider or a bee?"

They answer simultaneously—"spider, bee"—each positive he is right.

"Well, let me see the bite."

He holds out his dirty forearm. On the back I see a tiny mark. No swelling. No redness. "This?" I ask.

"Yeah, that."

"When did it happen?"

"About noon."

"About noon! You got me out of bed to see something like this? It happened at noon?"

"Hey," his friend calls out. "We're paying good money for this. We didn't come here to get insulted."

"Yeah," the patient adds. "We don't need this."

"There's nothing wrong with you," I shout. "And don't worry. I wouldn't think of sending you a bill." I stalk out full of fury and righteous indignation.

I suppose they had talked it over in a tavern as they drank their beer, argued about it, and finally decided the way to settle the quarrel was to have a doctor check it. They looked like laborers and must have led tough lives. Kansas heat can make an ordeal of summer work outdoors. I feel more sympathetic now. I wonder how they feel about the hot-tempered son-of-a-bitching doctor.

Sudden anger can destroy even long-standing relationships. Bonnie had many problems but was now hospitalized with mysterious epigastric distress. She was demanding and insisted on relief in a loud, querulous way. I had no explanation for her bellyache and other symptoms even more difficult. We had to rely on the cholecystogram for a positive diagnosis of gallbladder disease, and it was misleading sometimes. Bonnie's cholecystogram was negative and so, despite a strong suspicion that she was suffering biliary colic, I felt we ought to follow her rather than operate. Once she was better, I prepared to discharge her. Hospital census was high that week, so Bonnie was on the medical rather than on the usual surgical floor.

It was a Friday. I was off. My associate knew I had discharged Bonnie, but just before leaving she had another attack and on somebody's orders stayed in. He did not see her Saturday or Sunday. I did not see her Monday or Tuesday. In the middle of Tuesday afternoon, Bonnie called the office. Her message was simple: If I was not in her hospital room in five minutes, she would sue me for malpractice.

I flew to the hospital. Bonnie and her husband were furious at my neglect. I was furious at their threat.

We exchanged angry words. I felt coldly unconcerned with their problems. I resented the ingratitude, and said I could no longer work with them.

Later I learned she had gallstones. She relented enough to ask me to do the surgery. I declined, feeling rather mean about it. The angry exchange in her room that Tuesday afternoon had lingering effects. Though I no longer felt angry, I knew surgery would be too great an effort. If, as Origen believed, the purpose and end of creation is reconciliation, then Bonnie and I still have some work to do.

Money

Among the topics avoided in medical education is the love of money. Its importance is affirmed by our unwillingness to talk about it. But it erupts into medical practice willy-nilly and is part of the patient-doctor relationship. Art was a short, dark journeyman plumber whose wife died of breast cancer after a long illness. She was an appreciative patient, and we became good friends over the course of several years. Art was there as much as he could be, also grateful and friendly.

Art had diabetes and developed a blood-starved left leg that improved after my associate performed a bypass procedure. He was grief stricken after his wife's death and took poor care of the diabetes. One Saturday afternoon he was brought to the emergency room unconscious and with a large scalp laceration. The highway patrol said he had had an inexplicable rear-end collision with a moving vehicle on the open road. Art's right leg was hurting, too, and appeared pale and starved for blood.

I was assailed by a number of considerations. Was this a concussion? A fresh stroke? Could he have an intracranial clot? Might he have had an acute cardiac arrhythmia? A heart attack? Low blood sugar? And what about his damned leg? Where did it fit in?

We did not have in-house computed tomography scans at the time. Our practice was to follow the patient's neurologic status and refer if localizing signs appeared. I thought his painful leg was less important than the puzzle of his unconsciousness. My colleague would be back Tuesday, and by that time I felt the situation would stabilize sufficiently to permit an X-ray of his arteries and surgery. Art seemed to understand, though his leg hurt a lot. Something angered him, though, as he waited for definitive care for the leg. Tuesday arrived, Tom saw him and operated, fishing clot and debris out of his femoral artery and improving blood flow to his foot. In another month, however, the vessel clotted again, and Art had an amputation below the knee.

Then in an apologetic way, Art announced he was suing me. He was angry with one of our partners, but his lawyer insisted he had to sue me, too. "Somebody owes me a leg," he said.

Shortly thereafter an accusatory letter arrived from his lawyer. It was insulting and contained a peremptory demand for damages. Then the familiar waltz began. A consultant thought I should have referred him sooner. Art's lawyer threatened the malpractice carrier with immediate suit. The insurance company settled without asking my opinion, and I felt completely victimized.

When I protested, the representative said, "Well, it's our money."

"Yes," I stormed. "But my reputation." Come to think of it, it was also my money.

We sent a letter to Art telling him we would not be his surgeons in the future. All our interactions, conversations, affection became a pile of smoking rubble.

The arrival of laparoscopic cholecystectomy revealed that the love of money is not confined to patients and their lawyers. General surgeons have watched the domain of their craft shrink steadily for the past three decades. Orthopedic surgeons claim fractures and hand trauma. Ear-nose-throat specialists are doing thyroids and parathyroids. Maxillofacial surgeons claim the tongue and salivary glands, the larynx and epiglottis. Oral surgeons do fractured jaws. Endoscopists retrieve common duct stones. And so on.

That is why a threat to our claim on the gallbladder aroused such an abrupt and energetic reaction across the country. Be damned if they were going to take the gallbladder away from us.

Now, in retrospect, it is clear that laparoscopic cholecystectomy has a great advantage in reducing postoperative pain and speeding the recovery. True, we give up the chance to feel abdominal organs, and we do not control things as well as with open cholecystectomy. In the beginning, the risk-benefit ratio was not at all clear. But before it could be carefully defined, the technique was adopted by surgeons driven by publicity and patient pressure and, alas, by the love of money. In a confusion of terms, patients wanted the new "laser" operation that many presumed would be painless and risk-free.

Economic considerations helped precipitate the adoption of a technique that did represent real progress in competent hands, I believe, but that might not have. There was feverish and unseemly competition on the part of hospitals and surgeons alike to attract patients. Risks and disadvantages were glossed over.

So when I, finally climbing on the bandwagon, proposed laparoscopic chole-cystectomy to a young woman, I felt a real conflict. True, I had assisted on a large number. My assistant was skillful at it. But I had not done one before. Was I being fair to her? I explained the situation. She consented, and I did the procedure. Though I was anxious and sweating, it went well. It served my self-interest to do the procedure. But was it in her best interest to have me do it? This ripple of concern enters the relationship between all but the most self-assured doctors and their patients. There is always a better surgeon somewhere, a more experienced internist or obstetrician. If I am not the best, is it enough to be reasonably good?

Guilt and Absolution

Guilt is an ingredient of medical failure. One of the great defects in our peer-review system is that it makes no provisions for absolution. The legal system seems merciless, too. Mistakes in judgment and technique always seem unforgivable when looked back on. Certainly we knew better. Of course we should have checked for that bleeder or ordered that test or taken that precaution. The event casts a blinding light on our fallibility. We are tired, distracted, hurried, overconfident, careless, unprepared, or panicky and a patient suffers, perhaps dies. If there is to be healing, it has to come from the patient or family. The clucks of sympathy from one's colleagues fail to reach the very heart of the sorrow.

Glenda's mother was a strong old farm woman who presented with cancer of the left colon. I resected it. She had an uncomplicated course but complained of mild, vague abdominal pains for years afterward. I suppose I attributed them to adhesions. They did not disable her. She accepted the discomfort and lived with it. Then her pain changed character and became obstructive. I ordered a film of the abdomen. To my horror it revealed a steel clamp in her left gutter, large and brilliant against the softer shadows of her tissue. One powerful impulse was to hide the film. Yet her daughter Glenda was a nurse on the third floor. She would see the report. But another impulse was to be honest, not just because there was no other choice but because it was the decent thing to do. Were I Glenda's mother, I could forgive the clamp but not the deception about it. With my heart in my throat, I went up to her room and told her.

She and her husband and Glenda were wonderful to me. Their forgiveness was instant and unqualified. My relief was enormous, of course. But more than relief was involved. Forgiveness had an affirmative effect, a powerful strengthening of the bond of brotherhood between us. Their kindness and compassion enlarged my soul.

We operated the next day, found recurrent cancer in her abdomen, and removed the clamp that lay behind the colon we had brought down to the anastomosis. I have not forgotten that generosity about the clamp. It healed me when I could not heal Glenda's mother.

On another occasion early in my practice, I encountered an old man with a perforated ulcer. In those days I took the recovery of my patients for granted. So with little anxiety, I took him to surgery and sewed up the hole in his stomach. But he did not do well. I puzzled over his lack of progress for two or three days and finally reexplored him. His perforation had reopened. A couple of silk sutures had cut through the wall of the stomach and it lay open, dribbling bile-stained gastric juice into his abdominal cavity. I closed it impatiently with bigger sutures and another tag of omentum and just as impatiently waited for him to get well.

But he did not. His family showed increasing concern. I could not understand why. He just ought to get over a perforated ulcer. One evening I entered his room and found his family gathered there. I saw no reason for alarm. Nevertheless he took my hand. "Doctor," he said, "I forgive you. I know you did everything you could."

Well, I felt annoyed. Of course I had. Wasn't I an expert surgeon? I responded politely and assured him he would be getting well soon.

The next morning he died, no doubt of sepsis. Only then was the generosity of his act revealed to me—and the shallowness of my response to him.

Barbara was a piano instructor whom we were sure had abdominal carcinomatosis. She had been vomiting off and on, but her upper gastrointestinal tract showed no obstruction. I was not concerned enough to order a nasogastric tube preoperatively. Her surgery was scheduled late in the morning. It was a busy day, and the anesthetists traded assignments. As anesthesia was induced, I stood by her side. It did not occur to me or to the anesthetist to prevent regurgitation with a Selleck maneuver. Suddenly she vomited and aspirated. He quickly intubated and suctioned her, but the damage was done. After a miserable week, she died of respiratory failure. She was doomed with far advanced cancer but that made me feel no better. The aspiration added greatly to her suffering. I found it very hard to visit her when making rounds.

A month after her death her son sent me a note of thanks with a snapshot of Barbara. She stood near her piano and gazed into the camera with a joyful smile. Tears welled up in my eyes and gratitude in my heart. The patient-doctor relationship does not end with death.

Humor

Sometimes the relationship is full of humor. Lon is in his eighties, I guess. He could pass for younger. He is lean and likes to bicycle. Once a year he pedals from Riley to Clay Center to visit a cousin who is always horrified and urges him to quit. I believe he enjoys her expostulations about as much as the ride. Lon's hobbies include photography and gardening. But his chief delight is language, specifically polysyllabism. He will come in more for conversation than for anything serious. He has had a few little skin cancers, so I always check his skin. But he likes to josh me and Lylah, my nurse.

"Doctor," he will say with a perfectly deadpan manner, "I have inadvertently apprehended an epithelial excrescence prominently and progressively enlarging within the epidermal lamination which overlies the cartilaginous and osseous substructure of my olfactory protuberance."

Or, "If you will diligently investigate the pilar projections rising sparsely from the vertex of my cranial ossification, you will detect a macular callosity which may have malignant potential."

Some people, he complains, call him verbose, some loquacious, though he strictly limits verbalization to what is positively pertinent and necessary.

Laverne was a big, sunburned farmer who always brought a gust of cheerfulness in when he showed up for his follow-up exams after we removed a villous adenoma from his colon. It takes savoir faire to maintain dignity during a proctoscopy. Laverne was good-natured about it. During a procto one day, he told us about a recent adventure he and his lifelong friend ValGene had. It happened during the Iran hostage crisis. Feeling was high, and the presence of Iranian students at the college made some people uneasy, particularly, as it turned out, in the northern part of Riley County where Laverne and ValGene live.

That uneasiness escalated one morning when an abandoned automobile was found on a county road north of Riley. Someone—no one recalls precisely who—reported that two dark-complexioned males left the car and disappeared into the fields.

That night Laverne and ValGene attended a Swine Council meeting in Riley. The appearance of Iranians on the back roads of Riley County was the chief topic. By then, it was pretty well agreed that they were Iranians and probably terrorists. Folks felt pretty vulnerable. If terrorists could take an embassy guarded by marines, what was to prevent assault, hostage taking, and God knows what else in Leonardville and Riley.

About this time Laverne remembered his Japanese hand grenade. An uncle brought it back after the war and gave it to Laverne. When Laverne's aunt died, she left her farmstead to him, and Laverne, thinking of safety, decided to store the hand grenade in the loft of her garage. It occurred to him it would be a dangerous thing in the hands of a terrorist. ValGene agreed, of course. They agreed on just about everything.

So, when the Swine Council broke up, they piled into Laverne's pickup and headed for his aunt's abandoned farm. They parked and doused the headlights. Together they crept into the garage and up to the loft where to their great relief they located the Japanese hand grenade.

While they were looking for it, an elderly neighbor and his wife, returning from church, noticed the pickup in the shadows of the garage. Word of the Iranians and their abandoned car had earlier reached them through the grapevine, so, at the next crossroad, the old gentleman turned around. He told his wife to get into the back seat. Then he crept back toward what they supposed might be *them*, paused, noted the license number, and took off.

Laverne and ValGene, descending from the loft, noticed the suspicious slowing and accelerating of the passing car. Leaping into the pickup, they careened off in pursuit.

Laverne and ValGene were as determined to catch the terrorists as their neighbor was to escape. He told his wife to lie down in the back seat—he expected gunfire—and headed for Riley in a cloud of dust.

Laverne and ValGene could not quite head him off. The two vehicles roared into the sleeping community where the old gentleman pulled into a friend's driveway, doused his lights, and ducked. Laverne and ValGene lost him but went on hunting up and down the streets of Riley. The old fellow called the Riley County police department, reported his breathtaking escape and the license number of their maniacal pursuers.

It is safe to assume the police department was puzzled. Both Laverne and ValGene were respectable. They had a streak of fun and unconventionality, but chasing harmless old folks at high speed was totally out of character. Neverthe-less, the police checked with Laverne's wife, found her husband was, in fact, unaccounted for and when last seen was driving a pickup answering to the description furnished by the breathless old couple. An all-points bulletin went out even as the pickup lurched through the back alleys of Riley.

That accounted for Laverne's reception when he finally arrived home. His wife emerged from the front door before the truck stopped rolling and long before Laverne could launch into an account of his harrowing evening. "Now what have you done!" she demanded. "The police are looking for you!"

His proctoscopy was negative, and my day greatly improved by the story.

Affection

The sustaining force in the patient-doctor relationship begins with the doctor's affectionate commitment to the patient's welfare. A successful opera-tion is appreciated, but that appreciation can be transformed into fury if the surgeon is uncaring. If a surgeon is affectionate, friendship will spring naturally out of the interaction. Friendship works both ways and enriches both patient and doctor. It makes a successful outcome more pleasing, and it alone has the power to redeem tragedy.

Friendship takes care, though. It can become inappropriately intense, partic-ularly under the impulse of sexuality. I am not talking about the seductive patient or doctor. I am referring here to the surge of feeling that may hit a doctor or a patient in the necessary intimacy of the examining room. We read about instances in which overt sexual interaction occurs. Given the hungers and dissatisfactions of human beings, it is remarkable that it so rarely does. One reason, of course, is that a patient appears because of concern about a health problem. The mood is not romantic. It is my experience that sexuality evapo-rates when the complaint and treatment are the focus. Sexuality is a hurdle, and clearing it with the patient enriches the friendship with vulnerability recognized and respected.

The care of prominent or unusually wealthy or powerful people can be complicated by egotistic or financial temptations. Conversely, money and power can intimidate the doctor. They make me uneasy. Perhaps that is why I have found caring for a dying patient so satisfying. Ulterior motives are at a minimum. The affection is simple. Often it is all we have left to offer.

Teresa died of breast cancer. She helped found a support group for cancer patients that has met twice a month for the past seventeen years. When she became too weak to leave her home, the group came to her. She was very open about her faith and feelings. She simply could not accept trinitarian Christianity, although she was a loyal Baptist. Her belief in the mercy of the Almighty God allowed her this heresy and her gentle affection made it inoffensive even to the Methodist minister among us. Her husband died suddenly during the last stages of her illness, a cruel surprise that she was able to accept without bitterness. When her pain became too severe to control at home, she came to the hospital. A day or two before she died, she stopped me as I turned to leave her room. She looked directly into my eyes. She said she wanted to thank me for everything I had done. It was spoken calmly but with deep feeling.

We both knew this was goodbye. It was a fine moment, an act of surpassing affection. For her it was closure on the right note. For me it was a reward that renews itself each time I think of it.

Old Harry was about ninety. I had operated on him two or three times, and we always hit it off well. Prostate cancer and arthritis caught up with him. He slipped into a nursing home where I had visited him a few times. One fall afternoon I was called to the hospital where Harry lay in considerable pain with a perforated ulcer. We reviewed his options together. The following poem sums up the moment and the affection, which was painful.

> OLD HARRY
> But like broken redbud,
> just as dry,
> old Harry met his last catastrophe
> calmly, grimly,
> not unnerved by pain.
> "No surgery," he said,
> "I'm old. It's time to go."
> Then with real affection
> he took my hand and held it in
> the brittle branches of his own.
> Wounded by such fearless love,
> I yearned for shelter in the shiny hall.

The feelings of friendship are not confined to dying. I have practiced here for more than thirty-four years. The young man sacking my groceries had a complicated appendix. My friend in the office chair, looking up with quick interest, had a colon cancer. The young woman in Wal Mart—what a saga!—a survivor of multiple operations and hemorrhagic pancreatitis. She smiles a greeting, and what a history is in that smile! Frank is a retired veterinarian. In our kitchen, having returned a book, he rolls up his pant leg to show me how well he healed from the incision through which we evacuated a huge hematoma. He embraces me with tears in his eyes. He has heard about the recurrence of my prostate cancer. Such bonds are the fabric of community. To a large extent, they are the reason and the reward for a life in medicine.

I hope these vignettes suggest the variety and unexpectedness of the patient-doctor relationship. There are, to be sure, some constants: the doctor's desire to solve the medical problem, the patient's to have it solved as painlessly, quickly, and inexpensively as possible. But if we think about it in those terms alone, our mood gets overly serious and our conversation grows dull. Seen fully and without hindrance of preconception, the relationship between doctor and patient is the totally unpredictably richness one should expect from the encounter between incalculable, irreducible personalities. Often, the business of diagnosis and treatment is the least of it.

Chapter 4
A Deep Dying

JOHN STONE

In a letter written toward the end of her life, Emily Dickinson responded to a series of deaths among those she loved. She wrote, "The Dyings have been too deep for me, and before I could raise my heart from one, another has come—." In the fall of 1990, such a series of deaths began for me. The first was that of Jim Schwartz, who died on October 8, after a long illness.

I had known Jim for twenty-five of his sixty years. Born in Milwaukee, the son of a physician, he was educated at Swarthmore and received his M.D. from the University of Rochester. He trained in pediatrics at Yale, in neurology at Columbia. His wife, Phyllis, is a nurse. She and Jim have three children. Jim was professor of pediatrics and neurology at Emory; a consummate clinician, Jim's greatest satisfaction came from teaching. Students occupied a special place in his life, secondary only to his patients and family. Jim was also a devotee of classical music, a constant reader, an immensely literate man with a wry and joyous sense of humor. I do not remember ever seeing Jim without a bow tie, a sartorial touch that suited him perfectly. He was a short dapper man, with frontal balding, a ready smile, and sparkling eyes. Over the years, I came to admire his teaching. He and I first taught together in 1978, in a class on medical ethics for sophomore medical students.

Early on in his practice, Jim was confronted with those ethical issues that

34

inevitably arise when caring for young children: the neonate who weighs two pounds at birth and must struggle for life for weeks; the child born with a so-called neural tube defect, in which the spinal canal is open and the spinal cord unprotected, a condition that may lead to infection and paralysis; those tiny patients born with cerebral palsy or Down's syndrome.

With his large clinical experience—and unique personal attributes—Jim became a "doctor" in the best sense of the word (from the Latin *docere*, meaning "to teach"). The truth is, whether the subject was ethics or clinical neurology, Jim began to "teach" me while I was still in cardiology training at Emory. In that encounter, I was afforded an unnerving and close-up look at the art of his medicine.

In 1967, our second son was born—several weeks prematurely. Shortly after birth, he was found to have a perilously low blood sugar that announced itself in the form of generalized seizures. A prompt diagnosis of profound hypoglycemia was made and treatment was given. My wife and I were deeply grateful to the physicians and nurses who cared for him at Egleston Children's Hospital. At the same time, of course, we were concerned whether our son would have any lasting neurological effects arising out of this emergency. It was then that Jim Schwartz appeared on the scene. Fortunately, Jim understood intuitively that the treatment of any child must go hand-in-hand with the treatment of the child's parents. It was Jim Schwartz who watched our son with us, during both the ensuing two weeks of hospitalization as well as the long years of follow-up necessary to determine that he was neurologically normal (as he proved to be). My wife and I, then, knew Jim not only personally, but also as grateful parents. To us, he was a true "family doctor."

Jim Schwartz's own illness was diagnosed several years ago. As he prepared to leave on a trip to a foreign country, a routine chest X-ray was done. The report was disturbing: there was a mass within the chest wall, one originating in the myriad nerves of the region. It was the kind of tumor that may crop up in multiple locations within the chest, which is precisely what happened to Jim during the last few years of his life. The surgeon would open the chest, cut out all offending tumors he could find, then close the chest. Months or years later, the tumor would recur, not in the original location, but elsewhere. So Jim would have to have surgery again. In between these operations, he required repeated chemotherapy. Virtually none of his friends knew when he was having such treatments. He would simply check into the hospital, having mentally prepared himself for the severe nausea and vomiting he knew was coming. After most of the side effects of the chemotherapy had passed, he would return to work. Some of his colleagues learned that he had had chemotherapy only after his hair fell out completely. At one point, I ran into a completely bald Jim browsing in the university bookstore. Unconsciously, I must have looked askance at him. Smiling, he broke the conversational ice by introducing himself to me as "Mr. Clean" (the shiny-domed cartoon figure in advertisements for a household detergent).

A year or so after his first operation, Jim agreed, somewhat reluctantly, to come to my class on ethics and tell the young medical students what it was like to be sick, what it was like to be a doctor who was sick, just tell his story. Tell it he did. Many times after that class I wished that I had had a video camera running. The class was spellbound. His story was riveting, and I remember it in detail.

The night before his chest was to be opened, Jim told the class, the chief resident in thoracic surgery came by his room. He examined Jim hurriedly, then stood by his bed to talk for a minute. Jim could never get over what the doctor said next: "This is really big surgery tomorrow. You know that, don't you?" Jim was aghast. Not only was the doctor's remark not reassuring (especially on the night before surgery), it was insensitive, inappropriate, unnecessary. Jim was a physician, after all—he knew full well that the next day's surgery would be "big."

The surgery went well, Jim told the class. In the postoperative period, when Jim's chest was hurting with every breath, the surgical team would come by in the early mornings. Hurriedly, they would check the gurgling tubes coming out of his chest, look over the lab tests, divide up the work to be done. As they did so, they talked about his condition without ever talking *to* him in any but a perfunctory way. None of the surgeons, Jim said, ever asked him how he was feeling, then waited for the answer. There was only one person who did that: the physician assistant (PA) who worked with the surgical team. "That young man should have been a physician," Jim told the medical students. "He made me feel better just by coming in the room. He *always* asked how I was feeling—and he genuinely wanted to know. If I needed something done that didn't fall under the heading of 'usual duties,' he'd do it anyway. He'd prop me up on pillows, help me turn over in bed, get me a glass of water. He was incredible."[1]

After Jim's talk to the medical students, he responded to their many questions and comments. Afterward, in the unusually silent, sloping lecture hall, he and I sat and talked. I thanked Jim for taking the time to tell the class about his

1. Allow me to assert here that I have no wish to criticize in any way the post-op care rendered by Jim's surgical team. Overall, his care was superb. My intention, rather, is to underscore the special human attributes of this young physician assistant. Everyone in medicine knows that surgery can be a grueling enterprise, just as we also know that physicians can be among the most difficult patients to care for. It is to the surgical team's credit that they had the wisdom to retain this particular PA to work with their team.

illness. I told him that I had been moved by his story, that it was an important one for all doctors to hear, that I probably would not be able to resist writing about it. He smiled at this latter statement and gave me his blessing to try. I also told him my feeling that there was a striking literary parallel to his experience. It occurs in Tolstoy's masterpiece, *The Death of Ivan Ilyich*.

Ivan Ilyich is a high-court judge whose illness begins slowly, with a pain in his side, then crescendos until it is clear to everyone, including Ivan, that he is seriously ill (the illness sounds most like an occult, vitality-sapping, cancer). His doctors debate endlessly whether the origin of his trouble might be the bowel or the kidney. But as Ivan exclaims inwardly one evening, alone with himself and his pain, "It's not a question of a caecum or a kidney, but of life and . . . death." And so it was.

Consultants were called to see Ivan Ilyich, opium was administered, special foods were ordered for him. Ivan was dying, as he knew full well. Yet everyone who was supposed to be caring for him seemed to be merely carrying out their duties. Everyone except Gerasim.

Gerasim was a young peasant boy, a servant, who came in to tend to Ivan's basic needs. He carried out the chamber pot, helped him with the most ordinary activities of daily living—moving from bed to chair and back, for example—all those things that Ivan was increasingly unable to do for himself. In the course of Gerasim's ministerings, Ivan discovered that he was most comfortable, had less pain, when his legs were raised. The two tried putting Ivan's legs up on a chair, then added a pillow, but his legs were still not high enough for relief. Ivan asked Gerasim, "Are you busy now?" Gerasim said no, he was not busy, that he'd done everything that needed to be done for tomorrow except to chop wood. Ivan then asked him, "Then could you hold my legs up a bit higher?"

"Why, of course I can," Gerasim replied, and he did so: "Ivan Ilyich had Gerasim sit down and hold his legs up, and he began talking to him. And strangely enough, he thought he felt better while Gerasim was holding his legs. . . . After that, Ivan Ilyich would send for Gerasim from time to time and have him hold his feet on his shoulders."[2]

In the largest sense, Gerasim's ministering to Ivan amounts to not-so-simple human kindness, a therapeutic kindness that seems to me strikingly similar to that rendered by Jim's physician assistant. The acts of both arose out of what we call empathy. All of us know what we mean by the word *empathy*: we see it daily—or note its absence—in clinical encounters. But empathy may be difficult to define precisely. Most often, I like to use concrete examples to help me

2. Lev Tolstoy, *Death of Ivan Ilyich*, trans. Lynn Solotaroff (New York: Bantam Books, 1981), 88, 102.

define empathy. Or, because I am a poet, I use metaphor and simile to do so. For example, borrowing a term from molecular biology, I might suggest that empathy occurs when two people have the same "emotional receptor sites." I also like to think of empathy as being related to the principle, in physics, of "sympathetic vibrations." (Mount two tuning forks of the same pitch several feet apart. Strike one fork; then, with the hand, damp its vibration—the second fork will be heard to continue the original tone, even though it was not, itself, struck.) Thus, in an empathic situation, speaking metaphorically, two persons may *resonate together*: pain experienced by one person may not be *felt* physiologically by the other but may nevertheless be *shared*. Amid the technology of modern medicine, amid the rush-rush of the hospital, the beeps, blinks, and buzzes of innumerable machines, sometimes the most important thing we can do for a patient is to lift his legs. Or simply to listen.

Over the next several years, Jim did well, especially taking into account that he had several more operations on his chest followed by assorted chemotherapy. In fact, Jim had a total of six thoracotomies. The physician assistant rendered his inimitable post-op care in every instance. Despite these valiant attempts on the part of Jim's surgeons, the tumor always seemed to be lurking, always ready to recur. Then, Jim's bone marrow failed, a calamity undoubtedly related to his recurrent need for chemotherapy and its secondary assault on the marrow.

Thereafter, Jim was fatigued, anemic, short of breath. He required periodic transfusions of both red blood cells and platelets because his bone marrow was knocked out. His white blood cell count remained perilously low and overwhelming infection was always a threat. The possibility for a "bone marrow transplant" was raised. Jim said no, emphatically. His course continued inexorably downhill.

On October 7, 1990, the day before Jim died, I went by his home to see him. He lay on a bed in the den, his eyes closed, Mozart playing on the stereo. His daughter held his left hand. I took his right hand in mine. As I did so, Jim opened his eyes. He focused on me a minute, said "Hi, John. Thanks for coming." Then he closed his eyes again. Tears welled up and streamed down my face. I stayed with him for a while, then conferred with his wife, Phyllis. Someone in the family was having to be up around the clock, ministering to Jim's needs. Clearly the end was near. Phyllis had decided he needed to be in a hospital. I agreed with her totally. Later that day, Jim was taken to Emory Hospital in an ambulance.

Later, from Dr. Herbert Karp, a long-time mutual friend, I learned something of what happened to Jim that day. Herb had come by to check on Jim just as his stretcher was being wheeled into his room. Jim smiled weakly up at Herb and muttered, drowsily, "We just couldn't seem to manage to get this done at home." Within a few hours, though, Jim did manage to get it done.

Phyllis Schwartz asked me, Herb Karp, and two other physician-friends (Wytch Stubbs and George Brumley, the chairman of pediatrics at Emory) to take part in a memorial service for Jim a few days later. It was held on the Emory University campus, in a large church. Hundreds of people came. I gave some considerable thought to what my contribution to the service ought to be. At the time, I had just finished work on a long poem.

The text was written in collaboration with a composer-friend and destined to be part of a choral symphony that was to premiere in a few weeks. I decided to read the poem, which has elements of both celebration and mourning. From the pulpit, looking out over that vast audience, I maintained my composure well until I got to one particular quatrain from the slow *Credo* movement. There, just for a moment, my voice broke:

> Mourn for those who are no longer here,
> whose chairs are empty.
> Who sang their *gaudeamus igitur*,
> whose rest is silence.

Emily Dickinson was prescient, as poets have a right to be. For me, Jim Schwartz's dying was a deep one. From *his death* and from his life, I have learned a great deal about empathy.

I only hope those medical students were paying close attention.

Chapter 5
Travels in the Valley
of the Shadow

JOANNE LYNN

Introduction

A dozen years ago, I had the extraordinary good fortune to have to take an undervalued and academically meaningless job, having been assigned to a nascent hospice program and a largely ignored nursing home ward full of severely demented and disabled patients in long-term care. These were the least desired care settings served by a new geriatrics program. It was expected to be depressing and medically worthless work. Instead, it was wonderful. I have now served nearly two thousand persons who have died, nearly all in hospices or nursing homes. I have learned to cherish and sustain severely handicapped persons and those who provide care for them. That learning has relied critically upon participating in their lives and remembering their stories.

In telling real stories about patients, one finds that the telling is limited not only by the craft of the teller and the poverty of language in relating the complexities of human experience, but also by concern for the public exposure of private matters. It is not clear whether I should tell the stories of my patients, at least in ways that they can be recognized. Often the details that make the stories intelligible and important are also the details that make them identifiable. In telling these stories, I have disguised identifiers, including some less

40

important aspects of their stories. I have sometimes combined aspects of two cases. However, some who knew these patients will recognize them. I hope they will not find this objectionable.

Caregiving and the Professional Caregiver

One of the first responses I get when I tell people that I take care of people who are dying or permanently disabled and functionally dependent is that this must be depressing and unrewarding work. Not at all.

Paul Mastroianni was fifty-two years old and dying of a cancer of the neck when I first met him. His pain was overwhelming. His small frame, shrunk by the weight loss of extensive cancer, seemed even smaller as he huddled under the sheets afraid to move. His wife and adult children orbited the bed, nearly silently, faces drawn tight with the shared suffering. The hospice team embarked upon vigorous pain relief. His narcotic requirement was astonishing. Throughout, he was comfortable and communicative. When the drug administration was briefly interrupted or reduced, he was acutely aware of increased pain. His tumor grew, becoming larger than his head by the end, but we succeeded in ameliorating his pain.

More important, within the first two weeks in our care, his family relaxed and learned to trust that the terrible, life-dominating pain he had endured would not be allowed to recur. They no longer needed to orbit the bed, suffering with him. Instead, they redefined life as a family. They made his room the center of family life, bringing in meals, celebrating birthdays, announcing engagements, and sharing the hopefulness of awaiting a birth. A major part of the care team's discussion each week was what support was needed for this family's activities— use of the common room for a party, provision of supplies for meals, cosmetic covering of the disfigurement.

For the last few weeks of his life, he could no longer talk because of the tumor. Still the family life churned around him. One day, his wife and daughter erupted into argument. Another daughter commented to a nearby nurse, "Boy, that sounds like home."

The pregnant daughter began to consider having labor induced early so her father could see the baby before he died. After much discussion, she made peace with waiting for the natural course of events. During this period, I heard the family first talking of their faith. Although they had been practicing Catholics, it seemed that religion had been a ritual of their lives but that they were just discovering that their religious tradition interpreted and gave meaning to their current situation. This became more and more important, and priests and members of their congregation began appearing along with the family at all hours.

The baby was born and the grandfather clearly reveled in being given the pictures, which by now he could scarcely make out. But, there were complications and the baby was kept in the hospital for a week. We tried to pretend that there was no added tension, but we collectively held our breath. The patient was more and more somnolent, barely awakening to acknowledge someone trying to wake him up. Finally, the baby and mother came in. All of us were steeled for its being a most anticlimactic occasion. The patient by this time could not move his mouth except in a grimace, he could not raise his head, and it was not clear that he could see much except light and dark. The baby was put on his chest and pictures were taken. His arm came up and around the baby, his eyes opened and fixed on his daughter, and, as his wife related, "his eyes smiled." He fell asleep a few minutes later and died a few days later.

How can this work be other than rewarding? This family so obviously thrived, and this patient had so many good times in our care. When a physician operates to bypass a clogged artery or to fuse a dysfunctional set of vertebrae, it is uncommon to be quite so sure that good has been done. This family can look back on the good time that they shared under the shadow of death. The experience will illuminate and deepen their experiences over each lifetime. The caregivers involved can be confident that lives were made better by their efforts. What more can we ask of our work?

Emily Harding arrived at a nursing home with severe congestive heart failure. She could barely breathe, her color was a blue shade of white, her tiny body was weighed down with edema, and her family was frantic. An urgent series of telephone calls to past hospitals and physicians soon disclosed that she was expected to have died, having been found to have a cardiac ejection fraction of about 12 percent on an echocardiogram a few months earlier. The ninety-two-year-old Mrs. Harding had been living with her seventy-year-old daughter. The daughter had had a stroke and been hospitalized, and other family had arrived and decided on nursing home care for the mother.

After emergency administration of diuretics and narcotics, Mrs. Harding was briefly a little less troubled and the professional staff spent the next few hours getting to know the family, the patient, and the medical situation. An urgent care plan meeting settled on hospice care. She was expected to die within hours or days.

It was not to be. The reduced cardiac requirements of nursing home life and the reduced salt content must have fit well with the drugs we chose, and she stabilized. She returned to walking a little and enjoyed activities. She was just demented enough not to take offense and just cognizant enough to be bewildered by the new environment for a while. Then, it was just "home." We did no more tests, no more consultations, no more hospitalizations. But she lived and thrived for more than a year. Then she developed what seemed to be an aspiration pneumonia and acute pulmonary edema, which responded to diuretics and antibiotics briefly, but she did not regain strength and died within two days, comfortably. The family was at peace, as were the caregivers.

We were all surprised when the autopsy, which is routinely offered, found a large gastric cancer, metastatic to the lungs. One daughter expressed outrage that something so important could have been missed. "We could have treated that!" Her sister calmed her instantly by saying, "Yes, and we would have made her miserable." Indeed, one can hardly imagine that anything we could have done differently would really have improved her experience.

It is not hard work, in a way, and it is so rewarding.

Living Well While Dying

Ask anyone who is young and well what it is to live well and the responses will be predictable: productivity, wealth, comfort, friends, and so forth. While those things retain some value for those near death, my patients have forced me to accept much broader and more varied definitions of living well.

As a neophyte physician for a home care service, I went to see an octogenarian couple at home; Mr. Phillips with Alzheimer's type dementia had forgotten how to swallow. This I knew how to treat. I installed a feeding tube, gave instructions, and left feeling quite good about my skills. On the next day, I received a frantic call from the home care nurse. Mrs. Phillips had called nearly incoherent and crying and the nurse wanted me to come along to reevaluate what had clearly become a crisis situation.

Mrs. Phillips met us at the door and kept repeating that she loved Bill very much and would do almost anything that helped him, but that she had not been able to do what I had asked. It took a while to understand whether anything was technically difficult or whether there had been some adverse occurrence, like aspiration or vomiting. Nothing of that sort was the problem. Mrs. Phillips finally pulled herself together enough to look at me directly and say, "I just can't tie him down to our bed." Suddenly I saw the situation from her perspective. This man with whom she had lived for sixty years and whom she had tended during nearly a decade of mental decline was not really my "problem of nutrition and hydration" but her husband, lover, and spouse. Tying him down was not a mechanical solution to the problem of keeping a feeding tube in place, but a deeply offensive abuse.

In the discussions that followed, I also realized that taking him from home in order to place a gastrostomy tube was hard to justify for his benefit and contrary to the preferences of his wife. Seeing him—and her—in their home made it easier to see the impropriety of intervention. Letting him live as well as he had been living for as long as it lasted seemed to be the best course. He died at home some two months later. The only assistance needed from the "health care system" was an aide to help with a bath most days and occasional visits from and phone calls to the home care nurse. It makes me shudder to think how often we caregivers inflict terrible suffering as we thoughtlessly pursue correction of a physiological abnormality.

Sometimes the same blindness afflicts even symptom management. A fifty-six-year-old single woman with extensive local spread of breast cancer had been living at home alone until she became too disabled to change her own dressings or care for her daily needs. Miss Kauwalski was admitted to an inpatient hospice unit with erosive and fungating lesions from chin to groin.

The dressing changes were memorable. Every movement of a gauze pad caused pain. The odor and bleeding were unavoidable. She gripped the handrails of the bed with frail and bony hands, tensed her whole body, and moaned or sobbed. The nurses doing the dressing changes were reduced to emotionally exhausted shaking by the end. Yet the patient refused any pain medication. She did allow topical antibiotics to reduce the odor, and she was contemplative and communicative, with plenty of visitors. However, she would not explain her refusal to accept pain medications. We tried emphasizing that we could give short-acting medicines that would have little effect on alertness and that there was no problem with addiction. We tried bargaining with her to try once just to see. On this point, however, she was quietly firm.

Finally, after about two weeks of care in our setting, I sat alongside her bed and said, "Doing this to you twice a day is so hard for us. Is there anything you could tell me that would make it easier to understand?"

The answer that came back, after a long pause, was this: "What would we think of Christ on the Cross if he had been given your medicines?"

Miss Kauwalski identified her suffering with Christ's and, within her religious tradition (Salvation Army), the suffering that one bears during life is of value afterwards. Also, there is especially strong condemnation of the use of alcohol or narcotics within that tradition. At her funeral some weeks later, her friends eulogized her for her stalwart willingness to endure whatever God had in store and her avoidance of any use of narcotics.

Within her tradition and understanding, her choice was the only one that made sense. Once she shared it with us, removing our assumption that her choice had to be based on a misunderstanding, we were able to endure with her and to honor her commitments. Doing so was not easy, but doing so without understanding was almost impossible. Just as with Mr. Phillips dying at home without a feeding tube, working with this patient forced us to enlarge the scope of what could count as optimal care. Sometimes even profound suffering is not an appropriate target for treatment.

The Joy of Attending to Details

Millie Hardesty was fifty-three years old and dying of progressive maxillary sinus cancer when she was admitted to our inpatient hospice program. Independent and a writer, she was a kind and good-natured companion to all in her vicinity. Friends came by at all hours. They carried on extensive conversations, with her communicating by typewriting at great speed.

At first her cheek was sunken and her tongue immobile. Then the skin eroded, leaving a gaping hole to be covered with a bandage. Then the jaw broke, requiring supporting bandages; then the bone supporting the eyes gave way, leaving the now useless eye dangling into the space where the cheek once was. She was still alert and communicative, but gave up typing. It took us a few days to realize why. A care aide noticed that Ms. Hardesty winced and turned away when her useful eye caught a reflection in a mirror and also that the chrome band above the keys on the typewriter made a slightly distorted mirror.

Quietly and with only a nod acknowledging the patient's acquiescence in our plan, we removed the mirror and proceeded to tape over all reflective surfaces in the room—including the typewriter chrome and the flat surfaces of the hospital bed. The next day, after breakfast, she signaled for the typewriter, pointed to the work done, and typed "THANKS." Conversation with us and friends through the typewriter resumed and continued until a few days before death, when somnolence and lack of energy kept her in bed. I am sure that her renewed joy in life was as much a reflection of our attentiveness as of our action.

A distinguished black gentleman who had run his own accounting business came to inpatient hospice with a large suction tube through his nose and into his stomach, having been found to have gastric outlet obstruction from pancreatic cancer. Mr. Robinson said little but related that his doctor had told him that he would have this tube for the rest of his days and could never eat again. He stoically prepared to die soon and never complained.

I offered him the chance to try a period of time without the tube and told him that nothing very serious was likely to transpire, though he might vomit often enough to prefer that it be in place. He thought about this for a few hours, then called me to say he would like to try this course. Once the tube was out, we overheard him calling his sister to relate his joy at being rid of the noise of the suction. He said that the tube was not so bad, but having that noise with him for all the rest of his days was very disheartening.

A little later, I went in to offer him something to eat. Again, I told him that nothing serious was likely to happen—the worst would be vomiting. After thinking it over for a few hours, he called to ask if I thought he could have some orange juice. This was promptly brought and he sipped it for an hour. When I came to see him later, this very reserved man said, with a tear in his eye, "I thought I would never taste anything again." He spent his next ten days reveling in the enjoyment of small tastes of old favorites and the joy of nights of sleep unmolested by noise and tubes. He did vomit occasionally, but much food and liquid must have been making it through what must have become only a partial obstruction. Never did he have the tube reinserted. Again, a small detail, and the willingness to try an unusual course, allowed an unusual opportunity for joy, even in the shadow of death.

I am reminded of the story told to me by a chaplain. Alice, an elderly lady who was bedridden while dying, was left alone with her overly anxious sister Maude while others in the family were out. Maude persistently inquired whether Alice wanted orange juice, then tea, then sherbet, and so on. Finally Alice took Maude's arm gently and brought her to sit by the bed. Maude asked, "What is it, dear?" Alice answered, "What I really need is a tender morsel of juicy gossip." This story seems a particularly poignant reminder of the biblical admonition that man does not live by bread alone.

The Harder Cases

Nothing done by mere humans is always done well and the care of dying persons is no exception. Every once in a while, one encounters a patient who simply cannot allow himself or herself to be comfortable, or who stays hostile and angry despite all efforts by others.

One thirty-two-year-old woman dying of breast cancer complained of pain all of the time except when she was asleep. Her bitter whining about her discomfort probably reflected her anger at her misfortune and a lifelong socialization to expect others to take care of her, but we could find no entrée into her behaviors that allowed her to find peace and still to be awake, even though her disease would ordinarily have allowed this to be fairly readily achieved. Ventilating hostility, abusing staff, whining, or complaining did not help and time ran out before we really found a way to ease her anguish. As she became too weak to care, we brought her some relief, at least, with increased narcotics. In a setting where patient comfort and choice is so highly valued, the occasional patient like this is most disturbing.

The harder case, however, does not have anything to do with physical suffering. A substantial minority of patients who are comfortable but dying soon are simply weary with the waiting, finding that time has come to be without meaning. Perhaps this reflects our cultural dedication to productivity and goals, so that a period of time when no conventional goals can be achieved is rudderless. In any case, the young man dying of AIDS or the elderly woman seriously disabled by strokes might well ask, "Why bother?" Indeed, it is a difficult question to address. One looks to find something that still has meaning for the patient—an anniversary date, a family member's accomplishment, the realization of a long-awaited plan.

Once a seventy-two-year-old nursing home resident who had been quite apathetic and withdrawn and who claimed to find no meaning in living gradually grew more at peace and comfortable with herself. She was not the sort who said much and we did not know the meaning of the slight improvement in her enjoyment of life. One day I noticed that she always had her bed cranked up to just the same position when I came to see her. I stood so that I could see what she saw. Just outside the window, just out of reach of the lawn mower, was a group of large flowering weeds. A volunteer and I went to another place in the yard and found some more and set them in a glass near her dinner tray that evening. She smiled, patted the volunteer's hand, and said, "They are lovely, I have so enjoyed watching them grow this summer." But not all searches for some small meaning end so well. Sometimes there really is no adequate answer to the question of why to keep drawing a breath. Sometimes it seems that drawing a breath is merely a long habit, no longer worthy of being continued but also not important enough to stop. These existential, sometimes spiritual, questions are often among the most difficult conundrums in caring for the individual patient.

Bearing the Responsibility for the System of Care

Responsibility for the care of patients cannot end with the care of each patient. Each of us who participate in this endeavor also bear some responsibility for sustaining and improving a system of care so that it regularly and readily provides optimal care. How can that be done? In my experience, it has required some unexpected endeavors.

Patients ordinarily need a rapid response to their concerns. One way of achieving this, at least in closely knit, relatively small teams of caregivers, has been to train most staff to handle most issues nearly as well as the person conventionally designated as being in charge of that issue. Over time, in a stable team, this cross-training can allow nurses to know the pharmacology of analgesic drugs well enough to prescribe them, social workers to understand constipation and urinary problems enough to make a provisional diagnosis, physical therapists to understand dietary possibilities and concerns enough to provide advice to the family of a home care patient who is anorectic, and physicians to learn enough of the other fields to make referrals for services, give an enema, or adjust the length of a cane. This natural and helpful occurrence is sometimes caught in a harsh light when viewed from the perspective of acute hospital care. Nurses might be admonished for being so presumptuous as to propose a narcotics route and dose in a hospital, for example, although that would be expected in hospice home care.

Once a patient's body brought to the hospital for autopsy caused some furor when some of the paperwork was not in order. The chair of pathology called me to ask that we educate our physician group in managing these administrative matters. I assured him that I would review the issues with the social workers, which led to the comment that these were not matters for social workers. I responded that virtually all of our autopsy requests had gradually come to be made by social workers. This was a role that was unimaginable in the hospital but that was essential to optimal service in the home care and hospice settings.

Sometimes the obligation to establish effective systems of care leads one into unusual terrain. In the jurisdiction where I worked, the local interpretation of a federal regulation was that persons are not dead until pronounced dead by a physician who has examined them in person. Strictly speaking, a nurse at a patient's home or a nursing home was not allowed to tell the family that the patient had died or even to stop treatment until the physician arrived. Clearly, this led to ridiculous situations, unnecessary family travail and expense, and unreasonable disruption of the physician's other obligations. Despite no real opposition, success in passing legislation to ensure that certain nurses can determine that death has occurred took nearly eight years of lobbying.

Uninvolved observers often assume that those of us who like taking care of dying persons do so in part because we like to offer them control and choice among alternatives and would thus support allowing at least suicide, if not physician participation in suicide and active physician-supplied euthanasia. My commitment to care precludes this stance. My patients encounter a system that is dominated by concerns adverse to theirs. In our health care system, it is easier to get open heart surgery than Meals on Wheels, easier to get antibiotics than eyeglasses, and certainly easier to get emergency care aimed at rescue than to get sustaining, supportive care. In this setting, getting reasonable care often requires some struggle, usually with some advocacy by caregivers. It would be so easy to encourage dying persons to be dead rather than to find them services. If it were easy to get good care, the question of whether one should be able to choose to be killed would be troubling and important. But it is not easy to get good care. In fact, it is so difficult and unlikely that people might well seek death just because doing otherwise is so burdensome. Accepting a responsibility to work to change the shortcomings of the present system argues against reducing the pressures for change by removing the sufferers through death.

The Hardest Cases—Harms from System Dysfunction

The single most painful encounter of my professional life arose in the care of Faye Stills, a twenty-six-year-old woman with a lymphoma and diabetes. She had undergone a difficult course of surgery, radiation, and chemotherapy and had experienced a severe insulin reaction during treatment. The lymphoma seemed to have been arrested, though that was not entirely certain. She could moan, sometimes spontaneously and sometimes in response to discomfort during caregiving. She could not see, although she could hear at least loud noises. She could not swallow and drooled continuously. She was fed by a nasogastric tube, but was reliant on no other treatment.

Her husband was most attentive, seeking the best care and expecting that she would recover. Although he had already been told that it did not look likely, he simply did not register that possibility. Through nearly half a year of her illness, he had managed to keep going. He worked as a service station attendant, took care of their three preschool children, and came to the hospital. Clearly, he had not had a night's sleep in many months. When Mrs. Stills was admitted to inpatient hospice, he brought their children to see Mom for the first time since she had become ill. Naturally, they were a little frightened of this unresponsive shadow of the mother that only one of them clearly remembered. After a while, the five-year-old gently set about trying to wake Mom up. In the tears that followed for Mr. Stills, he seemed to acknowledge how hopeless that was.

The Stills family situation was complicated by an unusual feature. Shortly before Faye's illness, her aunt had died and left her assets to Faye. When the will was probated, Faye inherited about $20,000. She had deposited it in a bank in her name. Then came her illness and mental disability. The family was quite poor: no other savings, a little inadequate insurance, a rental apartment with three rooms, and no car. The certificate of deposit was their only asset, and no one could use it without court involvement, since only Faye's name was on the certificate. Yet, that certificate barred eligibility for Medicaid. It would have to be spent before she would be eligible.

As we came to know this family and their situation, we also came to realize that the lymphoma really did seem to be in long-term remission. Mrs. Stills was completely stable. She could live for many years in this state, for all anyone could tell. The only choice involved was whether to continue the feeding tube or not. I and my hospice team had discontinued tube feeding for a few such patients when the family related that this was the course most in accord with what the patient would have wanted, so we were willing to offer discontinuation of artificial feeding as an option. However, this case had two unusual features. First, having any reliable input from memories of Faye was unlikely, since persons so young rarely discuss how they will die and the course of the illness had been marked by such strong denial. Second, the conflict of interest over the money could complicate anyone's thinking about the situation.

Finally I sat down with Mr. Stills to initiate discussion of this issue. He told me how he saw the situation now, which included long-term survival in this severely brain-damaged state, and what he was worried about, which was mostly the care and well-being of the children. He mentioned that he needed to try to find some legal help to get access to the money so that he could pay for some regular child care while he worked. He clearly did not realize that Faye could not remain at the inpatient hospice indefinitely (although that had been said before). I told him that I had some concerns about the current situation that were shaped by certain facts about how the care system worked and began discussing the various elements.

I felt as though I were constructing a horrible medieval torment. First, Faye could live for years with her current plan of care. If that was what we decided to do, we needed to move her to a nursing home. Her assets would have to be spent first, then Medicaid would pick up the costs of care for the rest of her life. On the other hand, we could decide to stop the tube feeding, even though we expected that she could not take in enough nutrition or hydration to stay alive. If that was what we chose, we could expect that her time would be comfortable but also that it would be less than a month and would be spent in the hospice unit. This course would preserve the savings, as we would not seek to use that to satisfy the hospice bill. (Insurance paid part but not all of her hospice bills.)

Mr. Stills engaged fully in the discussion that followed, gradually realizing the terrible dilemma that faced him. He could help his young family past this terrible loss of his wife, begin to get past his grieving, and have some financial assets to help raise the children. This would carry the cost, however, not only of the usual emotional burdens about the propriety of forgoing life-sustaining nutrition and hydration, which are considerable, but also the concern that the course was chosen in order to save money. The other course doomed him and the children to a long vigil with an unresponsive wife and mother, not quite dead but certainly not quite alive. It spent their only assets in what seemed a largely useless endeavor. However, it did keep motives above question.

I left the discussion feeling profoundly weak and sad. It seemed outrageous for any community to arrange itself so that this situation arose. Surely, the community could let Medicaid pick up the costs without spending these small assets, or the community could require the assets to be spent for the children. It seemed so unnecessarily unfair. Much of life is, of course, unfair. But this situation was unfair and inhumane because human decisions made it so, not because the course of nature dictated that it be so.

Mr. Stills was put in agony by the situation he faced. He found a great deal of support in his church, although his pastor did not usurp Mr. Still's obligation to make the choices. Finally, he decided that he could not make peace with stopping the tube feeding, saying, "I just could never be sure I did it for her." She was moved to a long-term care facility, the money was spent, Medicaid started paying the bills, lymphoma recurred, and she died some two years later.

So often, such small changes could make the world so much better for dying patients. We have created a system in which meeting the needs of those who are disabled and dying is largely privately financed and only erratically available. When what a person needs is a reassuring, competent caregiver at the other end of the phone, available at any hour, that is not commonly available. However, the same person can get cataract surgery or hip replacement with no financial barriers. The system has been created to respond to the fears of middle-aged, middle-class men. Emergency rescue for a heart attack is freely available to all. Supper is available only to those who can pay for it, and to those who are both poor and disabled.

The Medicare hospice benefit is a troubling example. This national public benefit program should be required to be reasonably fair. It allows broad services to be offered in a coordinated way to certain dying patients. The package of services includes not only skilled nursing and medical care but also maintenance physical therapy, social work services, and medications. The coordination requirement assures that the hospice program shoulders the risk for unusually costly patient care needs and the responsibility for dealing with the annoyances of coordinating services. It is an extraordinarily good service for those it serves. Whom does it serve? Each program must have 80 percent of the patient days at home so inpatient days are used only for short periods to achieve symptom management or to give a family member a respite. Thus, persons without homes are not eligible, nor are persons with dysfunctional homes, nor are persons who do not have family who can be at home and unemployed for an indefinite period.

I made a home visit to a seventy-two-year-old Salvadorean woman who was dying of pelvic cancer and had recently been discharged from a hospital. Her apartment consisted of two rooms, with less than 120 square feet in each. There were six people asleep in those two rooms, and more than six children awake and active. The patient lay nearly unaware on a mattress in the kitchen. Roaches scurried along the dark side of the bed. A set of bite marks on her bare arm were probably from a rodent. Surely, if there is mercy in this community, she ought to be able to be cared for in a different setting. Surely there is a mandate to improve the situation for all of her family, but it is especially cruel to have to die too weak to chase off the vermin.

Hospice care also requires that death be exceedingly predictable. The requirement only says that the patient must be expected to die within six months. At no time in the debates over the enabling statute or in the later regulations was the exact meaning spelled out. Yet it is clear that a definition that encompasses only those who have a 99 percent likelihood of dying within six months is considerably more restrictive than one that includes a population that is anticipated to have a 50 percent survival at six months. Since hospice programs are at some financial disadvantage in long stays, the definition adopted has been mostly the more restrictive one. In fact, hospices generally average less than a month of care per patient.

At first, this sounds like a minor administrative issue. However, the entire issue of eligibility turns on this definition, and very few are eligible. Death from heart failure is difficult to predict, as is obstructive lung disease. Alzheimer's disease and strokes affect a person's life span in highly unpredictable ways. None of these etiologies is likely to make the patient eligible, no matter how sick or near death. More than nine of every ten hospice patients has a solid tumor cancer.

So, our major national commitment to improved care of the dying, hospice, turns out to be available, with only a little overstatement, only to those who have homes, families, some wealth, and convenient diagnoses. Although I served in both hospices and long-term care facilities for many years, it still troubled me greatly that patients dying in long-term care facilities had Medicaid benefits that provided only the care that barely escaped scandal, while those fortunate enough to have care in a hospice had all manner of personalized and attentive care. One should not be able to know these things and not feel an obligation to work for improvements.

Closing

It is an extraordinary privilege to have been allowed to travel in the valley of death with about two thousand patients. Dying serves to make life more precious and personal issues more pressing. Excellent professional care does make a difference in many lives, just as inattentive or inappropriate care causes incomprehensible harm.

We must find ways to ensure that new practitioners can learn these perspectives much earlier and be reminded of them more regularly. Perhaps medical students should learn to listen to stories like these from patients. Perhaps residents and young physicians should have to get close enough to dying persons to feel their suffering, to work within excellent care systems enough to recognize them, and to learn the skills and attitudes necessary to sustain a commitment to reform systems so that good care is more possible. We must also dedicate substantial effort to reforming the health care system so that everyone can expect to live well as they pass through the valley of the shadow of death.

Chapter 6
Letters of Intent

MICHAEL A. LACOMBE

I

Dear Rufus,

How marvelous the way you manipulate your doctors! I am *so* proud of you. You seem always to manage to remind them of their unhappiness. That is the epitome of style! Keep their profession a burden for them, and its heaviness will permeate every pore of their existence.

May I offer some minor points of technique?

The device of writing from Evil's point of view is not new. Mark Twain, in *Letters from the Earth*, used the technique masterfully. In this century, C. S. Lewis "discovered" a series of letters from a senior devil to his junior protégé on earth in his *Screwtape Letters*. In his preface to the book, Lewis acknowledged his own debt to an earlier writer, Stephen McKenna and his *The Confessions of a Well-Meaning Woman*.

The unique quality of what is to follow resides in Evil's intent to undermine particular *doctors* through his thorough knowledge of physicians in general. Whether readers choose to view the writer as Evil, Satan, the Devil, or fantasy, they would be well advised to remember that Evil rarely uses truth, unless the truth suits his purpose.

Portions of these letters originally appeared in 1989 and 1992 in "The War Within: I" (87:437–38) and "The War Within: II" (93:689–90) in the *American Journal of Medicine* (ed. J. Claude Bennett, M.D.).

54

Truth is always a good place to insert the knife. Doctors glorify themselves with their honesty. Wonderful! Keep your physicians worshipping Truth and they will have little time to worship anything else. That is, after all, the whole idea! But if you permit them to integrate truth into their very character, you will face disaster. This is a complex business here—the distinctions are very fine. Bear with me.

Some physicians, thankfully few, choose honesty as their way. Truth for them becomes a part of their nature. To say what is so is for them as natural as prevarication is for the rest. Keep your doctors always seeking some vague virtue they call Truth. Remind them of this; help them to make it their god. You can be sure that if they chase Truth as some impossible virtue, as an external cloak to clothe their pride, they will never attain it. Even in *this* frustration you will produce in them a measure of unhappiness. But there is greater unhappiness to be had.

Remind them of their patients. All doctors pride themselves on their honesty with their patients. Very well. Allow them to be blunt with their honesty. "The truth hurts," remind them. That sort of thing. Then deliver your masterful stroke. Permit your physicians to see—devoid of any empathy—the trembling anxiety they have caused with their honesty. Have them pity, if you can, the wretch before them, believing their patients to be *beneath* them and they, the grand physicians, *above* any such petty emotion. No person, you want them to think, would tremble before the Truth.

This is always a desirable line of thought, painted as it is with tones of noblesse oblige. Permit them a brief, condescending Kindness, which they immediately see in themselves and for which they are quietly and humbly proud. Now insert a brilliant change in their thinking. Whereas before they have been blunt, even cruel, with their honesty for the sake of Truth, now you will have them deceive for the sake of Kindness. In their Kindness, they will hide the truth, manipulate, evade, *even lie*, "for the good of the patient." How Mephistophelian! Help them along. Feed them Wisdom from the Ages, some Emily Dickinson perhaps:

> Tell all the truth but tell it slant.
> Success in circuit lies.

Their patients will surely sense the falsehoods, mistrust your doctors, become, we hope, their adversary, and add to their yoke of unhappiness. If their patients do not appreciate their efforts, they will reason, it is only because they do not comprehend their Kindness.

There is a danger here of which I readily warn you. Be careful, lest they, in a momentary lapse, identify with their patient, sense a oneness with this other, and in a surprising display of charity, ruin your game with their compassion. Keep them feeling guilty if you can—because pride follows guilt—and keep them always contemptuous, of course.

Next, work on their relationships with their colleagues. All physicians suffer guilt and so are ripe for criticism. Very well! *Use* this! Cultivate in your doctors a critical nature, then have them believe it to be the best sort of Honesty. If they are critical, if they joust and jab their friends, why it is only because they search for Truth, and that is a hard road, tell them. Doctors love hard roads. Maintain in them a healthy arrogance. They are "better," if only by a little—"above the fray." That is the idea.

They are never to be kind, of course. Blunt honesty is preferred. That is "the way of the scientist," tell them. Doctor to doctor, tell them—person to person.

Do you see how this erodes their relationships? Not only will they begin to *believe* their criticisms of their colleagues, but they will suspect that their colleagues engage in similar condemnations of *them*, and so they will mistrust them. Litigation is of great help in this confusion. Our legal fabrication of discovery is a marvelous invention! Any confession your physicians make to their colleagues, any commiseration, the slightest comfort from them is *discoverable*! There can be no sharing of like concerns therefore, and no solace—only a vapid isolation. And ask your doctors, while they are in the dock, whether perjury sins against truth or their Truth? Help them to find the answer.

Hospital business is a great ally as well. Use it to your advantage. Remind them, in this age of prospective payment and capitation, that honesty costs money, that the government has their patients in thumbscrews, that therefore cheating the government is always a virtue. Maximize payments, get away with something, tell them. American society will assist you in this business. If government cheats its citizens, so, it is widely believed, citizens must realize it is their duty to cheat in return. (Lying is always easiest when done for the higher good.)

Keep your physicians mired in this confusion. Sometimes their patients will be "the higher good" and at other times, their hospital will be so. You may need to prompt them to lie for "the good of their patients," distorting a diagnosis or the severity of an illness, and so forth. At other times you will encourage them to modify medical records for the fiscal soundness of their institution—again, an appeal to this higher good. Never must they begin to believe that these laws are unsound and their government decadent and uncaring, or they may attempt to do something about it! They must never begin to take action. Better, advise them, to "fight fire with fire." Point out to them that, as always, two wrongs *do* make a right.

You will want to perpetuate this confusion of truth in your physicians' dealings with their families. They will be "absolutely honest" with them as well. In this case, they will either glorify or denigrate their profession, never, of course, telling their families how it *really* is. Make them role models of discontent for their children. Why should *they* be happy? Then remind them about patient confidentiality and about the need "not to bring their work home." This will isolate them further. You do not want them talking to their spouses, and least of all, feeling from them any measure of understanding. Their arrogance will help you here, of course. They are *the doctors*, remind them, and must never appear weak or in need of caring. *They* will do the caring. Use their pride too, with their families, to lay down the law, to tell them how it *will* be. They must never listen carefully to their families—they might hear the truth. Keep them busy, then, and full of their own importance, racked by demands, and you need never fear this.

In the end, they will lose touch with reality. They will lose their very selves! They will begin to tell the truth *as they believe it to be.* Their arrogance will fill them with conviction. They will wonder who they are, what they are about, and where they are going. They will pose as the skeptic, the fashionable iconoclast, the philosophically critical professional—the agnostic in vogue. With this loss of themselves and with their isolation, you will find it easy to get them to lie and believe it to be true.

Anytime you find them sitting quietly, holding a hand, exercising compassion, attempting to tell the truth, try to get them to look at themselves. How grand they are! How compassionate! How honest! Lose them in their Pride. Return them to rumor, innuendo, gossip, and evasion. When your doctors seem to resist, give them a dose of the Immortal Bard to bolster them!

> Take note, take note, oh world!
> To be direct and honest is not safe.

A little of this will go a long way with your doctors, I assure you.

Good luck next week in court. I will keep watch.

Yours sincerely, Belial

II

My dear Rufus,

I am so delighted in how you torture your doctors. This whole area of emotion is such a marvelous attack point. Distance your physicians from their feelings and your game with them is won. To create in them a state wherein they are wholly and completely out of touch with themselves, wherein they are so detached from any genuineness of emotion that any honest feeling will appear as an affectation and be discarded as such, is the perfect solution for our purposes. Replace any emotion with *attitude*, always appealing to reason. That is their soft spot. We have talked about this before, remember. They are never to *feel*. Whenever you can get them to *think*, to *intellectualize*, in preference to *feeling*, you will have them closer to our camp. I will give you an example.

Suppose your doctors have made some brilliant diagnosis or embarked upon a course of therapy producing unparalleled success. They have, shall we say, achieved a victory of sorts. They will naturally begin to feel joy. Permit them to develop this emotion and they may begin to be *happy*, may even enjoy their profession for its own sake, may relish their role as doctor, may *like* what they are doing.

You do not want this.

Any man or woman who enjoys a pursuit for its own sake while at the same time disdaining any notion of ulterior gain is disgusting to us and worse, in danger of being lost. At all costs it is your job to prevent this. And what have I told you is your primary instrument in cases like this where you must separate your pigeons from their humanity? Why their pride of course! There we are. Permit them to be *proud* of themselves, *proud* of their brilliant diagnosis, *proud* of their miraculous therapy. The more lavish, the more unctuous, the more self-indulgent the pride the better. Allow them to talk about their achievements—the grander the better—present their accomplishments at Grand Rounds, compare themselves to others, even write about their breakthroughs. They must contribute to the literature, tell them. Make them work at it, chew on it until it becomes a tired quid of tobacco in their mouths, and as tasty. That is the trick. Make the mere thought of these accomplishments turn their stomach. Then you will have them.

Do you see what this does? Instead of the joy of accomplishment, instead of a pleasure in helping others, as *He* would have your doctors feel, you permit them just enough insight to see how pompous they are, and so allow them to doubt themselves for it. Delicious! The good deed becomes disgusting, distasteful to them, and, we hope, something ultimately to be avoided. Anyone can do *that*, they think. The literature is full of *that*, they say. Why should I bother?

You say you have doctors of pretense already? Perfect, my dear Rufus, perfect! Give them no insight into their arrogance whatsoever. They consider it a virtue, would you believe! Allow them simply to continue on into this realm of self-indulgence, on to the committees, on to the learned lectures, to the business end of medicine, never to return to their original source of fulfillment.

The practice of medicine is so replete with opportunity for emotion that it could be potentially dangerous for us, my dear Rufus, were it not that your doctors and the vast majority of their colleagues are so ready to pervert that emotion, so *eager* to do it I must say, that their field of endeavor becomes for us a wonderful opportunity. Take, for example, the emotion of sorrow, of sadness. Let us examine that for a moment. Medicine is so replete with opportunity for it. It is positively sickening! There is cancer and consumption, palsy and plague, children with leukemias and elderly pensioners reduced to demented fools. Allow your doctors to suffer with their patients and you risk losing everything. Attack them on many fronts here. Allow me to instruct you.

First, keep in them this attitude: these, their patients, are The Great Un-washed—simply inferior—for which, to which, upon which they perform their *business*, often just for *money.* Never permit them the merest glimpse of camara-derie, never allow them for one brief instant a notion of kinship. You want your doctors to consider their patients as mere children, although never letting that prejudice reach their consciousness. These are fine points here. Pay attention. You want in them the sense of entitlement similar to that with which we endow our good friends, the priests and ministers, who serve their *poor children* of the Third World. The more your doctors think of their patients as inferior, the more you can cultivate in them the sense that they are helpless children, or even, we might hope, higher animals, the less likely they will ever feel sorry for them or empathize with them. Disease just *happens* to them, they think. It is *their* due, *their* condition, a part of life, at least, they reason, a part of *their* lives.

A second way to attack any possibility of empathy is thankfully already being done for us and without, I must confess, very much direction from us at all. Medicine was, you remember, historically a *man's* profession, and so there developed within the profession that *men*, and therefore doctors, should not feel for their patients, should not cry, should never allow that note of sadness. It would affect care, so the argument goes, get in the way of things. Their univer-sity professors still openly teach this stance, both in didactic measure and through example. Physicians must be objective, devoid of any feeling. Care for their patients, yes, but in a paternalistic way, as one cares for children or, ha, barnyard animals. This attitude, which is so devilishly succulent as to seem to have been planted by us, continues all through the young doctor's training. Patients are talked of not as people, but as *cases*, as in this *cancer* on Ward 23 and that *infarction* in the intensive care unit, this *leukemia* and that *lymphoma.* Death becomes an unfortunate result, a negative response. Delightful! It is so hard to feel empathy for data, for an item of research.

There is a third way to attack this emotion of empathy, this sense of profound sadness for the plight of humanity, and one must often turn to it. (But never, *never* underestimate the power of this emotion, and its ability to do us in.) If all else fails, if your doctors begin to feel sorrow for their patients, begin to sense the common bond He would have us feel, very well, *allow* the emotion. But *pervert* it! Turn it to pity! Let them smell the fetid breath, the rotting flesh, the melanotic stool. Let their stomachs turn at the mere thought of gangrenous tissue, perforated bowel, atrophied brain. Permit them to see their patients as simpering fools, helpless wrecks of humanity with whom they could never identify. Let this pity grow, spread like a cancer within them, and you need not worry.

There are other emotions to pervert, my dear Rufus, and you must pay attention to them. There are all of the emotions akin to love, for example, and they can be very dangerous in medicine. Fortunately, doctors will readily assist you in these perversions. There will be the usual sort of bootlicking and pandering you can imagine. Have your doctors look within themselves for the ulterior motive, the secondary gain, the possibility of advancement, power, prestige, money. Now you have reached the turning point for your doctor-fools, my friend. Either permit them to persist in this line of thinking (allowing them to term it pragmatism, self-knowledge, or even—ha!—honesty) and we will have them indeed. Or, barring that, let them see this admiration for another as really nothing more than filthy greed, and they will soon stop this foolishness.

They may observe the nurses and other doctors about them, see their capacity for emotion, their boundless empathy, their tenderness, their patience, their identification with the suffering, and so develop the deepest of feelings for these other individuals. Dangerous territory here. Unless you are careful, Rufus, a genuine unselfish love (that disgusting *agape* sort of thing) will develop. Approach this sort of love as you would any other, Rufus. *Pervert* it. Convert it to lust. Help them focus on their feelings as sexual, help them act upon this male-female thing they feel, this simple manifestation of their own biology, so natural in itself and nothing more. Fill their hearts with lust. Render them then unlovable. Wonderful!

They will love their patients as well, but here the fertile field of psychiatry will help you a great deal. They can easily be made to believe that these feelings are nothing more than displacement, transference, or some petty neurosis best left unidentified.

We have talked before about managing your doctors vis-à-vis their families. It is worthy of repetition here. The more arrogant they are toward their families, the more they see their family members as patients too, as meddlesome, as common, as rife with problems as the rest of them, the better off you are. From their families they will only get complaints, and a further extension of their tortured days. No happiness there for them. They will not want to stay at the office, and they will not want to go home. How delightful! What is left for your doctors then? Why, the usual mirages of life: money and the material traps it will bring, and lust and its juicy entanglements.

If at the end of the day your doctors feel utterly drained, unrewarded, "burnt out" as the saying goes, you will have done your day's work. Never let them leave the office with a skip in their step, a smile in their hearts, an aching for the new day.

The desired result in your doctors, Rufus, is this: they will reach the end of their career not having enjoyed one minute of it. They will suffer one emotion and one emotion only, that of enmity. They will spurn their patients, they will detest their colleagues, they will scorn their mentors, and they will slight their families. They will damn Love and their notion of it and become hollowed by their enmity and neither know what they are thinking nor how to feel. They will despise themselves. They will die confused, bitter old people.

And they will be yours.

Happy hunting.

Yours, as ever, Belial

III

Idiot colleague!

I will be direct! You are in danger of losing your simpering fools!

What have I been telling you? Do you think I undertake these difficult letters to you for mere folly or better, for self-aggrandizement? *Why* have I talked to you about feelings, about emotion, about compassion? Because I *enjoy* that slop from above? Must I feed you your instruction as pablum roughly shoved in the fool's gaping mouth?

Very well, bumbling moron:

You will *lose* your doctors through empathy. You *win* them by attacking empathy. Could anything be more simple? And, as with anything else, what is simple to you, you make complex for them. *There.* Can that sink into your addled brain?

How could you think that if you permitted your pigeons to feel empathy from another, you would not lose them? What are you thinking? For Hell's sake you might have stepped in as soon as they had felt this compassion, this sappy, cloying pap from that whimpering fool. You could have had them see it as pity, condescension. It should be elemental, Rufus, when working with doctors, one always has a head start. How many times must I repeat that?

Even in their premedical years, these young doctors have a delightful touch of intellectual arrogance that can be such a joy to work with. Without any help from us, a specialness, a sense of entitlement creeps in, before a life experience—or literature, always a danger to our work—can twist and deform this delicious character we so desire. They are easily enthralled with physical chemistry, differential equations, and physiology, disciplines they can hardly turn to in the bleak years of middle age when they sense, but do not know, that we are closing in.

Doctors gain entrance to medical school by besting their fellow beings, rather than through understanding them, receiving such lavish praise that a sharp sense of knifelike competition becomes alloyed with their character. Already here, at this moment, the game can be won, if you will only use your head. Secretly they believe themselves to be superior, even at this juncture, while openly pretending compassion. This is the sort of division of mind and soul we strive for! Develop this dichotomy, and you will have your people. They will be Eloi to your Morloch, your Tess, your Jude.

Reflect on what you have accomplished so far, Rufus. Your doctors have suffered residency. Their training has been something that was *done* to them, neither a happy time nor an experience blessed with a single measure of human understanding. It was a time for which they must seek retribution. And seek it they will, if you will only *let* them, exercising greed, lust, pride, envy, and any other of those admirable attributes for which we so love humankind.

But *you* permitted them to feel empathy from another! More about this later.

Here is what you have in your doctors. They are both highly trained and poorly educated. They cannot feel, and more important, they scorn feeling. They believe themselves to be thoughtful individuals, a belief that we encourage, when really their minds, if they could scan their scope, are filled with slogans, jargon, hype, opinion. They are usually wrong but never in doubt. They can hardly think their way out of the most simple conundrum.

Young doctors are people who invent words, mnemonics, acronyms, and actually pride themselves on doing so, who lose the meaning of words, and by station, by title, or by mere strident voice, hatch for themselves a life's philosophy.

Take, for example, this "empathy," a quality you yourself, Rufus, seem to be oblivious to. Your doctors believe that *empathy* is no different from *sympathy*, is simply a romantic delusion, or merely an intellectual understanding of another's feelings. It is their decision, after all (they believe), to define it however the term seems to fit—much as *virtue* has, I might say proudly, come to mean only *chastity* and has been rendered devoid of any hint of wisdom, or prudence, or courage, or integrity. Their definition, their "thinking," they quietly believe, is superior to that of Plato and Aristotle, who are so dated these days and unread by doctors anyway. We *love* this sort of thing. Rufus, it is not even incumbent upon you to place these thoughts in their heads. They are *there*. You must merely encourage them.

Lack of empathy they call "clinical hypo-competence" and list several precise steps designed to attain that competence, an approach that has worked so well for them in organic chemistry. Their students in turn recite their mentor's formulae, believe they, too, are empathetic and move on to the next event. Some will even ask if empathy is really necessary for the scientist-physician of today. Such doctors will variously be called forward-thinking, iconoclastic, ahead of their time and will spend their time basking in this adulation. Such a wonderful example for others! *They* need not talk to patients, need not touch them. They *image* them, *scope* them, *cath* them, "work them up," as might a computer.

Your own doctors are well on that road. Let them continue.

But now we come to your own grave error, Rufus.

Your doctors have lost patients, "allowed" them to die, they believe. They feel guilty for their death, responsible for it, to blame. They have missed something. They were not thorough enough. They did not stay late enough at night. There were tests they did not order. They might have obtained another consultation. They should have performed another procedure, ought to have sent the patients elsewhere. These are *healthy* emotions Rufus. We *like* this sort of thing.

And what did *you* do? You permitted them to talk to others about their feelings! And not just to any other, but to the *nurses*, and not just any nurses but the nurses who were caring for their patients. Idiot! Did you not see that the nurses shares the doctors' feelings and therefore must understand. Could you think that the nurses, *especially* the nurses, would be devoid of compassion in this circumstance? *Of course* the nurses will understand the doctors, *of course* they will sympathize with them, *of course* they will weep like a common peasant, *of course* they will hold each other devoid of any healthy, wholesome sense of lust, sex, and degeneracy.

Will you listen, Rufus?

Should this happen again, remind the doctors gently of how strong they are and of how strong they should remain. Nudge them toward the isolation they have come to know, sprinkle it lightly with a dash of arrogance, add pride, and a healthy disdain for this *touchy-feely* stuff they scorn. You will avoid similar danger in the future. If they persist, if they must seek out someone to talk to, by all means have them turn to those experts in clinical hypo-competence! Themselves devoid of any emotion, these experts in empathy will help your doctors recognize that they are in the presence of a strong feeling, will define that feeling for them, categorize it, help them "deal" with it, offer support, and lead them to the welcome distraction of biostatistics and grand rounds.

I will not lie to you, Rufus, though I am tempted to do so. Having once experienced these connections with others, with these sniveling sobbing wrecks of humanity—these nurses—they will likely seek them out again when the going gets rough. You must remember our cardinal rule. *Corrupt this encounter.*

The next time, the nurses will be open, less guarded. The doctors must see that as vulnerability. They will reach out to each other. You must help them see this as a sexual invitation. Invite them to admire each others' bodies rather than search each others' eyes. Allow them a brief moment of insight, of utter disgust for themselves that even in this situation, they are still, only, sexual animals. The nurses will offer compassion. The doctors must see it as pity. When the nurses weep, the doctors must see it merely as weakness. When the nurses talk about their loss, their love for the patients, their connectedness with those patients, the doctors must think only disparagingly of the nurses' emotional involvement and their deplorable lack of objectivity.

What you do, Rufus, in other words, is just change the focus a bit. The nurses are exercising their true feelings, their emotions, placing your doctors at risk of connecting with that. And so, instead you have the doctors judge the nurses, treat them as objectively as possible, as patients in other words, as they have been so thoroughly trained to do, just as they treat coworkers, colleagues, and family. The doctors will then turn from the nurses and pity them. And you may then rest more easily.

While we are on this subject of empathy, let me review two other points.

The first is the notion of misplaced priority. This is quite an easy matter with doctors and hardly bears mentioning here. By now you have had a brush with failure, Rufus, and nothing should be beneath you. In common with lawyers, politicians, and academics in general, doctors have conflicting demands, and they share with these other professions the notion that since the demands are on *them*, they are all therefore equally important. Because *they* are important. And since it is *they* who are being asked, *they* who are omnipotent, they can never say no nor judge the priority of the demand. Consequently there is never enough time and too many demands, none attended to adequately. Meditation, contemplation, intellectual (and emotional) debate are notions they will "get to someday." Your doctors are academics after all, and you may enjoy this edge. And I must admit, I am following one full-time practitioner who so styles himself as doctor-banker-economist-priest-socialite that I am continually tempted to sit back and leave the driving to him.

The second facet of your doctors' lives is more complex, less easily understood by those of our students who struggle with this critical point.

Experience and emotion are our enemies.

They can destroy any hope of eroding not only empathy but also integrity, character, prudence, courage, honesty, professionalism. In the area of emotion, you cannot hope to wipe clean any and all emotion from your doctors who are, after all, human. That is a fruitless endeavor and foolish besides. All love, all positive feeling, all sense of closeness becomes lust, or greed. Simply that. Any feeling of what others may term "honest" anger may be lumped together with disappointment, pique, and resentment under the heading of aggression. Find an acceptable term for any positive feelings and file those feelings under that term for your doctor. I have found that most doctors like "approval," as a comfortable condescending "emotion" with just the right touch of noblesse oblige. There you are. Three emotions: greed, aggression, approval. They hardly need more than that.

Experience comes to doctors in many ways. But you need not worry very much about their talking to patients. The proceduralists, the imaging department, and their eager students insulate them from any patient contact and will nearly accomplish your work for you here. Still, be careful. Make any case presentation concise, emphasizing the facts, the science, and leave out the soft stuff, the family history and social history, and the disgusting analysis of the patient's reaction to illness. By all means do not allow this presentation to be at the bedside, a rarity these days anyway.

In the realm of experience, the worst sort of danger for you resides in the appeal of literature for your doctor. The two standard approaches to this threat are still very reliable. I will review them for you, then offer you a third, novel approach, a favorite method of mine. First, doctors pride themselves more on being scientists than on being artists. Play on that. Scientists read nonfiction, the drier, more scientific, more devoid of experience and emotion the better. Artists are thought soft, undisciplined. Stories are for schoolchildren.

The second basic approach to this problem resides in the concept of misplaced priority and time-pressure we have discussed above. The world's greatest literature (as you will help your doctors to believe) is of such a high priority that one must devote a special moment for it. Let them buy the books, Rufus, let them stack them in the corner together with their old journals as something that they will turn to someday, will study someday, may write about someday. They may even believe, to our delight, that they will teach such literature in their retirement. They have, of course, lost the true art of thinking and confuse purchasing the book and possessing it with having read and understood it. You will find them ready to deceive themselves and others on this point. They will be asked at cocktail parties if they are familiar with such and such, and you will hear their ready answer.

Never worry, Rufus, about the busy doctor turning to literature or philosophy or religious thought. Their thinking is so distorted, so jammed with the buzzwords of the day, that they could no more sort their way through Kierkegaard than they could return to the membrane biophysics that was deemed so important to them in their formative years.

The third method, my own, is rarely employed, and then only for those clients of ours who are in the best of times most difficult. Should you come upon physician clients who *read* literature and who actually seem to enjoy it, put into play those aspects of their character you are familiar with, those that will quickly strangle this decadent behavior. They are competitive—very well, permit them to believe they are better than Dostoyevsky. Since they are the scientists, are judgmental, analytical, ever-questioning—let them read books suspiciously, wondering about the author's hidden agenda and the author's real intent, looking for the moral, then have them disagree with what the author supposes it to be.

Finally, even in reading literature the doctors must set priorities, and you can help them misplace those priorities here as well. They *will* read great books? Turn them toward a philosophy of despair. They must get the intellectual "feel" of the twentieth century, tell them. Little experience and narrow emotion— those are the keys, Rufus. At any rate, give them more questions than answers, if read they must. Remember, by now, think they cannot.

Finally, a word about poetry. Never, Rufus, never permit your doctors to understand poetry.

Yours, Belial

Part Two
The Teaching of
Empathy

The secret of teaching is not to bring empathy to medical practice but to keep it there despite the rewards of technology. In this part, the writers suggest how medical students can retain their empathy, even enhance it, throughout their training.

Harold J. Morowitz, one of our few Ph.D contributors, finds the problem in his experiences as a member of the medical school admissions committee at Yale: *empathy* has been a code word to imply that the prospective student is intellectually inferior but not a complete disaster. Far more important than character—to the selection committees—are the grade point average, the MCATs, and an absolute commitment to science. Physicians' character, personality, and attitudes are formed during their college and medical school training, Morowitz avers. He leaves me feeling that more exposure to literature would give some impetus to empathy during the torment of medical training.

The sole nurse contributing to our book, Jeanne LeVasseur, writing with David R. Vance, describes the fluid boundaries between medicine and nursing. LeVasseur finds empathy to be attention to the individual patient, an understanding of how any illness can be a threat to the person: empathy is a mode of caring, and primarily an emotion. I interpret them to suggest that the physician should not view empathy as a tool. This brings to the fore the question of how much empathy has its origin in the patient and makes irrelevant the question of whether empathy can be objective.

Shimon M. Glick has his own plan for integrating humanism into the "one legitimate school of medicine, and that is scientific medicine." Good physicians must gather *all* the necessary data; for them the personal history is as important as any biochemical profile. With "reverence for life" and the "awe of the human being" that are essential for empathy, the compassionate, mature physician must also have a stable worldview. For Glick, religious values and a sense of duty are compelling components of the compassion that leads to empathy. He offers an account of what is done at Ben Gurion Medical School to turn students into compassionate, empathic physicians.

Richard L. Landau attributes to me a dichotomy to which I make no claim: "When science triumphs, the humanities are the losers." Firmly rooted in science, he praises scientific medicine for bringing a scholarly approach to medical practice making it possible for physicians to cure, not simply care for, their patients. A liberal education may be helpful to the scientific physician, he agrees, but its place is in college, not in medical school. On the importance of imperturbability, he agrees with Osler; others may worry that even if an imperturbable physician can set a broken leg or calm a stormy thyroid, in the rage against death—or sorrow—an aloof expert giving advice without passion might not seem so caring. The world Landau describes is so gray and cold that alternative medical practitioners will surely beckon patients to their sunnier clime.

Richard and Enid Peschel provide one key to bridging the gap. Science is essential to empathy; it is not "either-or," it is "and." Dr. Grenvil in *La Traviata* was the good physician *before* science transformed medicine; empathy is both restricted and enhanced by scientific knowledge. In the vanguard of those who have transformed "mental illness" into "neurobiological disease," and "psychiatric" problems into "brain disease," Richard and Enid point out how antiquated notions of "mental illness" lead to "selective empathy." Too many doctors who can share the pain and anxiety of a cancer patient will treat the schizophrenic with disdain, if not fear. For them, as for Glick and Landau, to provide modern empathic effectiveness, a physician must first understand the scientific and medical problems at hand.

I concur with that comment: to be truly ethical or empathic, a physician must first get all the data, must be sure to understand the scientific background of the "case." To help requires knowledge; an ignorant doctor is truly unethical. But for the good doctor these spheres merge; the good doctor looks at all aspects at the same time, swinging into the spirit and the mind, as well as the body of the patient. Even death may not always come as a defeat; sometimes, just sometimes, it may come as an answer to life, and the empathic physician must recognize that time.

Stanley Joel Reiser describes how classifying patients by their diseases lessens empathy. However valuable for the discovery of defects in the body, technology blocks the physician from the patient. The physician sees the body and not the person, with the result that patients see less of their physicians and more of the technicians who scan their organs. Reiser repeats Morowitz's point, that the student-teacher relationship is where empathy is nourished. Transmission of knowledge alone, but not of attitudes, lessens empathy. How an institution fosters its staff and students, how instruction is carried on in the classroom or clinic, what can be called "collegiality," establishes life-long patterns of behavior and thinking. Alas, our students are not educated in empathy but in precision. The history—what some call the narrative—is so hard to duplicate that it fades in importance, along with the patient who gives it. The ability to enter into the life of another is the essence of empathy, but it is far more difficult than breaching a sphincter. Reiser closes with an ethical code for teaching that deserves close reading.

H. M. S.

Chapter 7
The Pre-Med as a
Metaphor of Antipathy

HAROLD J. MOROWITZ

Being a member of the Yale Medical School admissions committee was a strange job for a Ph.D. whose research on biogenesis can only relate to the health professions via the most remote path involving 3.9 billion years of evolutionary history. Yet a curious series of decisions had me seated across a desk from an earnest medical school applicant from one of the big three Ivy League schools. He seemed like an admissions committee's dream candidate: a biochemistry major, he had a 4.00 grade point average as well as substantial independent research experience.

Yet at the end of the interview I found myself giving him a very low rating. His very self-assured and highly intelligent answers showed a disjunction with the questions that had been asked. In short, the applicant knew what he wanted to say and did not hear the questions or the interviewer's comments. He had a very low E.Q.—empathy quotient—and I reasoned that if he did not hear the interviewer when he was in the very vulnerable situation of being interviewed for medical school, then he would surely not hear what his patients were going to say when he was no longer vulnerable but they were.

All applicants accepted to the Yale Medical School receive two independent interviews, and the case in point was no exception. The second interviewer was a faculty member in one of the clinical departments who gave the applicant a very high rating. In cases where a candidate receives two very different scores, a third interview is routinely offered, and its assessment in this case agreed with the very high rating.

The student was accepted, but he chose to enroll in a different medical school that must have also been impressed with his credentials and presentation. Although I have no problem in accepting the collective wisdom of committees in such cases, I did emerge from this particular case wondering about how important my clinical colleagues regarded empathy as a qualification for medical school and for the practice of medicine.

This story suggests that the subject of this book might be considered from the point of view of the undergraduate experience. I suppose that over the past thirty years I have counseled on the order of 500 students wishing to discuss a career in medicine. No one has ever asked, "Do I have enough empathy to be a health professional?" Hundreds have asked, "Do I have high enough grades in organic chemistry or high enough MCATs (Medical College Admissions Test) to get into medical school?"

Indeed, I have a little secret to tell. Back in the 1970s, when admissions were perhaps at their most competitive, empathy and compassion were the unspoken code words that writers of letters of reference would use to indicate that "although the candidate is not up to academic standards, I think he or she might nevertheless make it as a physician." A colleague of mine once asked, "Do you have to be academically second-rate to have those human characteristics we would all like in physicians?"

Medicine is different from most careers in that, for the majority of aspirants, a committee decision made in one's senior year in college determines whether or not one can pursue this career. The key to that decision is: grade point average, science grade point average, mark in organic chemistry, MCAT score, extracurricular activities, and letters of recommendation. And to achieve high marks, an incoming seventeen- or eighteen-year-old undergraduate must have made a firm decision to pursue a career in medicine or be disadvantaged by every fluctuation from absolute commitment that is part of the normal undergraduate experience. There is thus a certain alienation between premedical students and the rest of the undergraduate body, whose critical choice point comes later in life.

Premedical students with a firm goal in mind are of course aware that they are in an extremely competitive situation, and being smart people they compete—hard. This often scares their classmates. I have known students to rearrange their entire schedules to avoid those sections of undergraduate physics that are largely peopled by pre-meds. If you doubt that these students feel alienated, I would also tell you of other students who spend most of four years not revealing to their friends that they are planning to apply to medical school. These folks clearly have empathy with their classmates, but at the price of honesty.

Since the admissions process drives the undergraduate experience, and the undergraduate experience would appear to be negative or neutral with respect to empathy, it seems prudent to inquire who and what drives the admissions process. By describing the steps between the undergraduate applicant and the medical professionals on the admissions committee, we can explore how these steps may influence the undergraduate development of future physicians.

Medical School Admissions Process

The requirements, I assume, are set by faculties of medical schools, with occasional unsolicited help from state departments of higher education. The assurers of the requirements are faculty admission committees aided by a bureaucracy of admissions officers and their staffs. These bureaucracies interact with pre-med advisory committees and various officials at undergraduate colleges up to the level of deans who administer the application process. Note that the majority of these officials are not themselves medical professionals and may in certain cases exhibit antipathy toward that profession.

In addition to standards and qualifications, the admission process is dominated by paper. Because of multiple applications and the ease of copying, I would conservatively estimate that nationwide more than five million pieces of paper are involved in application and assessment. This is on the order of twenty-two metric tons of paper, most of it dense with information. As a result, methods are sought to efficiently process the paper and to discourage low-yield applications.

The information overload encourages functionaries at every level in the admissions process to turn over work, and thereby decision making, to individuals below them in the hierarchy. The response to vast amounts of information also leads to great reliance on numerical assessments such as grade point averages and MCAT scores. In other words, show me a student who has a 3.95 GPA and MCATs in the upper few percentiles and does not exhibit overt sociopathic or pathological behavior, and I will show you someone who is going to be admitted to medical school regardless of subtle personality factors such as sense of empathy. Thus the initial triage decision is mostly numerical in its basis and is made at the secretarial level of the admissions committee under the director of admissions.

Very often, the full information on an applicant does not reach the admissions committee, which relies on premedical committees at the colleges to provide a preliminary filter. This applies particularly to letters of recommendation which, under the best of circumstances, would offer the best window into the applicant's personality. Very frequently the letters are submitted to the undergraduate service which then abstracts them and sends a summary recommendation to the medical school. The more thoughtful premedical services send copies of the originals along with the summaries, but even when this occurs, the summaries have a significance out of proportion to the letters of recommendation because of paper overload.

The summary writers thus play a major role in determining who gets accepted to medical school. The members of premedical committees at major universities are usually undergraduate science faculty, physicians from the university health service, and occasionally members of the medical school faculty. At smaller universities, the committees are largely science faculty and members of the student counseling bureaucracy.

At the major research universities, many of the science faculty are rather contemptuous of students who elect the M.D. route rather than the Ph.D. route. At the next level of university, some fraction of the science faculty took the Ph.D. route because they were unable to get into medical school. Thus the individuals who are mentoring premedical students may themselves lack empathy for the medical profession.

These premedical committees often place grade point limitations on the applications they will service, which again shifts the decision to an easily administered number, and away from less quantifiable evidence.

A synergistic relationship often develops between the premedical committees at the colleges and the admissions bureaucrats at the medical school. Thus, summary letters may be written in a code both parties understand. As I have noted, I suspect the phrase, "This individual possesses a keen intellect and has done a fine undergraduate research project" would be taken positively, whereas the phrase, "This individual is deeply compassionate and has a keen sense of empathy" would often be translated as "I'm having a hard time finding something nice to say about this individual."

Pre-Med Course Requirements and National Exams

Among pre-med course requirements, a special place is reserved for organic chemistry. I have not been able to determine the reason for this or when it emerged as a requirement. Clearly it must have been after the 1910 Flexner report, when undergraduate science requirements were instituted. I suspect that Emil Fischer's classical studies on sugars, amino acids, and nitrogenous bases must have convinced professors of medicine of the important role organic chemistry plays in understanding the human body. In addition, Paul Ehrlich's discovery in 1910 of the usefulness of Salvarsan in treating syphilis established a bridge between the chemical industry and medicine. As pharmacology and biochemistry emerged at the core of medical studies, organic chemistry came to be required as a sine qua non for medical studies.

Two difficulties emerged over the years. First, the courses in the chemistry department were oriented toward training synthetic organic chemists rather than physicians and tended not to engage the interest of premedical students. Second, a tradition arose in chemistry teaching that resulted in a very tough grading system. Since there are more pre-meds than chemistry students, organic chemistry classes tend to have a large proportion of pre-med majors. As a result, organic chemistry tends to be a competitive class. I have often heard students refer to organic chemistry using names such as "Sadism 101." Frequently, students take organic chemistry in summer school at a college other than their alma mater. If the grade is too low, they do not claim transfer credit and take the course a second time. I do not know why organic chemistry is taught with so little empathy, but untold numbers of students have voiced this complaint.

The one step in the undergraduate training process that relates directly to compassion is the hospital volunteer work that is frequently an extracurricular activity of premedical students. Very often this experience as a volunteer helps to build empathy with patients. Since it is known that admissions committees like this type of activity, however, many undergraduates view it as a requirement, and when thus viewed, it provides only the illusion of compassion. The intense level of competitiveness perverts even the best of motives.

I next turn to national exams, the MCATs and the growth industry of cram courses designed to prepare people to take these tests. Although these exams and the courses to prepare for them heighten the sense of competition among pre-meds, they do nothing to enhance their empathy for patients or their plight.

In my more than forty years in premedical education, I have found very little that is designed to foster empathy and much that serves to isolate premedical undergraduates from those humanistic pursuits we would identify with empathic ideas. While we all like to think of medicine as a vocation or a calling, the undergraduate experience has the character of a rat race with little positive reinforcement of those characteristics that will humanize the relationship between physician and patient. Those premedical students who emerge with personalities that do know how to humanize physician-patient interactions have learned that skill on their own.

Solutions

One senses we are once again drifting toward the two-culture problem so forcefully stated by C. P. Snow in 1955. One of the little-known replies to Snow is Aldous Huxley's essay "Literature and Science." Huxley draws a distinction between science, which develops a highly specialized jargon to express public knowledge with great precision, and literature, which deals with expressing the inexpressible—those inner feelings that force the author to struggle with the language to communicate with the reader yet with understanding and feeling. Empathy is surely more closely bound up with literature than it is with science. This suggests an approach to humanizing the undergraduate pre-med experience: a course on literature and medicine that explores the doctor-patient relationship. A few works that come to mind are *Arrowsmith* by Sinclair Lewis, *Code Five* by Frank C. Slaughter, *Five Patients*, by Michael Crichton, *Out of My Life and Thought*, by Albert Schweitzer, and selected poems by William Carlos Williams.

This proposed course in medicine and literature is indeed a modest approach to the problem of humanizing the undergraduate premedical experience. A much more thorough evaluation of medical school requirements and the undergraduate experience are necessary if we are to fundamentally improve the doctor-patient relationship. I would suggest that the time has come to reevaluate premedical training in light of the enormous changes that have occurred since the 1910 Flexner report. To be specific, I would suggest a National Research Council study undertaken under the supervision of the Institute of Medicine and funded by the National Center of Research Resources of the National Institutes of Health. How's that for a precise suggestion? I would hope that such a committee would consider the effects of the four formative undergraduate years on the personality and attitudes of the emergent physicians.

Chapter 8
Doctors, Nurses,
and Empathy

JEANNE LEVASSEUR
AND DAVID R. VANCE

What can nurses teach doctors about empathy? Nurses feel they have a great deal to say, for empathy and caring are the cornerstone of nursing. Moreover, caring is part of what distinguishes nursing from medicine. But don't doctors care about their patients? It seems almost an indecent question, insulting and preposterous to imagine otherwise. Nonetheless, nursing as a profession has historically been concerned with empathy and its place in the patient-caregiver relationship. A scan of a medical bibliographic data base, which shows more entries on empathy in the general nursing literature than in the general medical literature, offers evidence of nursing's continued concern with this issue.

Many nursing theorists define nursing with reference to a principle of care. For example, Donna Diers has written: "Nurses observe, listen, test, assess, diagnose, monitor, manage, treat and cure. But above all, nursing is caring. As a profession we have any number of divisions among us. . . . But the one thing upon which nurses agree is that the essence of the practice, and thus the knowing, is caring" (Diers 1990, 41).

Professional knowledge—for nurses—comes from caring. Diers continues,

"Nursing, practically alone among the human service professions, deliberately tries to train its young in empathy, sensitivity, and compassion (ibid.).

Shouldn't medicine attempt to train young physicians in these same qualities? If medicine has historically emphasized the development of scientific knowledge and technology over the understanding of patient needs, a new emphasis appears to be emerging. In 1983 the American Board of Internal Medicine advocated the teaching of humanistic qualities to internists (American Board of Internal Medicine 1983). Some medical schools have developed programs that use trained lay people to play the role of patients, to improve students' interviewing skills (Stillman et al. 1983; Stillman et al. 1990). At the same time, nurses' functions have begun to look more like those of the traditional physician. From the perspective of her eighteen years as a staff nurse, Theresa Stephany comments:

> Comical though it must sound today, in the '70s nurses did not routinely carry stethoscopes, much less use them for anything except blood pressures. . . . We were neither educated nor expected to listen to breath, heart or bowel sounds. Physicians started and managed IVs; central lines did not exist, nurses did not draw blood; there was no Amphotericin B. Only the head nurse spoke to the doctors; hyperal was done in the ICU we gave IM Demerol every four hours, PRN for terminal cancer pain; MDS pushed what rudimentary chemo existed, and, even in our worst nightmares, we could not have imagined AIDS. . . . Today's nurses wear scrubs and athletic shoes and own the finest stethoscopes for a reason. (Stephany 1992, 4)

As both nursing and medicine evolve, there is a possibility that outdated conceptions of their respective roles will be perpetuated. Certainly popular opinion accords nursing the empathic role of understanding the patient. Nursing distinguishes itself from medicine in claiming that it cares for the whole person rather than focusing on disease. As Diers has written, "Doctors are authorized by the states to practice medicine, which is to diagnose, treat, prescribe and operate—on disease, not people. Everything else is nursing (Diers 1990, 39).

As a society, we regard the roles of doctors and nurses as complementary: physicians traditionally diagnose, order tests, and manage treatment, while nurses tend to patients and the environment of care. In an earlier era, Virginia Henderson, an influential nurse, wrote poetically of this: "The nurse is temporarily the consciousness of the unconscious, the love of life of the suicidal, the legs of the amputee, the eyes of the newly blind, the means of locomotion for the infant, knowledge and confidence for the young mother, the voice for those too weak or withdrawn to speak" (Henderson 1960, 4). She advised that the nurse must "get inside the skin" of her patients to know what they need. Many would say that this is a fine expression of empathy, that is, a transposal that allows a person to step into the inner space of another, to help.

But what of physicians? If nursing distinguishes itself from medicine in its focus on empathy and care of the whole person, then haven't physicians lost something, at least in the public perception? The bad press physicians have received in the last decade has centered on their relations with patients (Cousins 1985; Engle 1977). "My doctor doesn't listen to me," grouses patient after patient. One study found that when patients recount their problems, they are interrupted by the physician approximately eighteen seconds after they begin to speak (Beckman and Frankel 1984).

Many will argue that with regard to empathy, the physicians's role is different from the nurse's. The physician makes objective decisions based on physical findings, laboratory data, and the patient's symptoms. Emotional detachment is necessary in order to consider patients and their problems objectively. Some will concede, however, that empathy, made concrete in the exercise of listening skill, might facilitate obtaining the medical history and thus contribute to diagnosis and even management (Bellet and Maloney 1991). In this view, empathy is regarded as a tool that the skillful physician might employ to render a better diagnosis.

Doctors and nurses differ in their views of empathy, one seeing it as a technique, the other as caring, even as they become more involved in the technical aspects of caregiving. Physicians have also spoken of the difference between medicine and nursing in this way. Barbara Bates wrote that "the primary role of medicine comprises diagnosis and treatment—the 'cure' process. . . . In contrast, the primary role of nursing lies in the 'care' process, expressive in nature, and consisting of caring, helping, comforting, and guiding" (Bates 1970, 129).

Still, as health care has become more complicated, nursing has held fast to its principle of care, perhaps knowing that it cannot be abandoned even in the face of technological and scientific advance.

Nonetheless, professionals of both fields have struggled with the fear that getting too close to patients will impair their professional judgment. Nurses were advised to cultivate an emotional discipline with regard to their patients, but also to avoid becoming hardened (Melosh 1982, 58). One nurse recollects, "We soon learned that we could not be nurses of calm judgment and steady nerves unless we detached ourselves from the personal element in every case. . . . This does not mean we were callous to human suffering but rather that we sought to relieve our feelings by skillful help rather than through emotion" (ibid., 60). William Osler too advises the young doctor that no quality is more important than imperturbability, though he also warns physicians not to harden "the human heart by which we live" (Osler 1904, 7).

As empathy might impair professional judgment, it is easy to imagine that it belongs more to nursing than to medicine. But as care has become more sophisticated and technical, nurses have learned to grapple with objective science and analytical modes of decision making just as physicians do. Consider the independent roles of nurses in intensive care units, clinical nurse specialists, and nurse practitioners. Here especially, the roles of physicians and nurses have become blurred, a reality that both professions need to recognize. Nurses are no longer as distinct and different from the doctors as they once were. This has implications for the concept of empathy. For the present, nurses still claim a special interest in the issues of empathy and caring.

Perhaps a question for the future is, if nurses are going to become more like doctors, will doctors also become more like nurses? But more important, what are the contributions empathy makes to practice? Aside from facilitating human relationships, and contributing to interviewing skills, is empathy even necessary to expert practice? Or does it, as some claim, distract from objective decision making? We believe that empathic understanding is basic to expert practice for both doctors and nurses.

The Standard Conception of Empathy

The word *empathy* entered the English language as a translation, after the Greek *emátheia*, of the German *Einfühlung*, a word coined by Theodor Lipps in his discussions of aesthetic experience. A less artful English rendering might be "feeling into." Empathy is generally thought to be a process or event by which one perceives and understands the subjective experience of another person. Empathy is regarded as a mode of perception in contrast to the more "scientific" observations of objective testing and knowledge. The standard idea of empathy retains a clear implication of immediate and subjective perception that yields understanding of the private, inner experience of another person. For many, empathy involves a psychic transposition in which the empathizer temporarily leaves his own subjectivity, as it were, and enters that of the other. In an early influential discussion, Robert Katz wrote that "when we experience empathy, we feel as if we were experiencing someone else's feelings as our own. We see, we feel, we respond, and we understand as if we were, in fact, the other person" (Katz 1963, 26).

Other concepts abound. The process of empathy includes "a kind of vicarious experiencing; the empathizer 'tastes' the other person's experience" (Zderad 1969, 660). "When a person empathizes, he abandons himself momentarily; he relives in himself the emotions and responses of another person (Ehmann 1971, 72). In 1975, the influential theorist Carl Rogers stated that empathy involves ". . . entering the private perceptual world of the other and becoming thoroughly at home in it (Rogers 1975, 4). Rogers went on to say that "to be with another in this way means that for the time being you lay aside the views and values you hold for yourself in order to enter another's world without prejudice. In some sense it means that you lay aside your self" (Ibid.).

Such characterizations of empathy persist. In 1991, Bellet and Maloney wrote that empathy is "the capacity to understand what another person is experiencing from within the other person's frame of reference, i.e., the capacity to place oneself in another's shoes. The essence of empathic interaction is accurate understanding of another person's feelings" (Bellet and Maloney 1991, 1831).

More sophisticated recent analyses of empathy (Davis 1990; Gallop et al. 1990) characterize empathy as a multistage process that includes stages such as "crossing-over" or "matching" that are strikingly similar to the earlier notions of empathy itself.

One reason that these characterizations of empathy rely on metaphors of telepathy is that their authors want to discuss a form of personal relatedness that involves more than cold intelligence, something more than mere observation, understanding people in their individuality, apart from general features described and classified as a case. Subjectivity is just the sort of thing that cannot be objectified; it seems natural to infer that a full understanding of the subjectivity of another must elude not only measures of public testing and verification, but also any full and literal conceptualization. General conceptualizations will never be adequate to the understanding of persons, for they can never match the variety and subtlety of inner personal experience, and so feeling more than thinking gives the life and color of human meaning to our intellectual comprehension of others.

Katz argues for a conception of empathy that bridges the subjective and objective. He conceived of empathy as an intuitive perception arising from "subjective involvement" but then aimed to retrieve this mode of perception for scientific knowledge by attaching a component of objective detachment.

> Empathy consists of feeling. It involves the inner experience of feeling oneself to be similar to or nearly identical with the other person. There is an important distinction between simple empathy and the use of

empathy as a technical and specialized cognitive technique. Both simple or raw empathy and empathy as the tool of the scientist are capable of yielding objective information not attainable through ordinary rational and intellectual techniques. When empathy is used in a professional way, it becomes more consistently effective, more versatile, and more penetrating. With discipline, empathy or "empathic understanding" becomes a fully reputable scientific technique. (Katz 1963, 26)

Such discussions are motivated by a concern that a caregiver's expertise be used in conjunction with genuine care for each patient as a human being. The motivating fear is that caregivers, however brilliant their technical competence, may fail their profession by not really caring, perhaps because of burnout or worse because technique blinds them to the humanity of their patients. In either case, the feeling-cum-understanding called empathy provides the needed supplement to technical knowledge.

For all its emphasis on feeling, sensitivity, and caring, the standard conception nevertheless still posits an *active observer* and a *passive subject:* one person observes another and gains information about the other by using a technique. The observer sets aside self and prejudices, relives, tastes, or reexperiences the other's experience from the inside, and then withdraws to reflect on the experience. This way of thinking about empathy presents the empathy theorist with a dilemma: either empathy is a subjective process and what one learns can be neither described nor verified, or it is a method by which objective knowledge of a special sort may be retrieved. On the first alternative, it is not clear that one learns anything, and on the second, empathy is a technique that may be alienated as much as any other technique from the motivations of care. For all its promise, the standard conception of empathy does not illuminate the essential connection between knowing and caring. It is stymied by its presupposition that a person is fundamentally divided into a *mind*, characterized by subjective, private inwardness, and a *body*, available to objective, scientific knowledge.

Empathy as Understanding

The human understanding that we wish to indicate with the word *empathy* is not so much a psychological transposition as a respect for, and openness to, the concerns of the patient whose benefit is the entire aim of the caregiver's profession. The idea of empathy that is truly crucial for clinical practice is that of genuine attention to the individual patient's concerns, and the acceptance of those concerns.

The good served by the caregiving professions is a human good that finds its value within the daily weft of concern and hope that forms the fabric of any human life. Every *profession* forms its knowledge, both theory and practice, in service to such practical human value.[1] Interest among health care professionals in the topic of empathy signals the special character of the human value to which their professions are a response.

The idea of empathy is important for the caregiving professions because illness is a threat not just to a person's interests but to the very possibility of having interests of the sort that make a human life worth living. Unlike other professions, the main goal of the caregiving professions is the amelioration of suffering (Cassel 1982). Cassel defines suffering as the perception of "an impending destruction of the person" (ibid., 640); for him personhood is not just by a human body or a subjective inwardness, but by a complex of social rules, identifications, and relationships. Physical illness can undermine a person's ability to function as a parent, spouse, friend, scientist, artist, or citizen. Yet these functions and their meanings are the very sources of the self, the basic integrity in need of protection when illness occurs and medical intervention is necessary. Physical illness can threaten the constitution of a person and cause suffering.

Cassel argues that not only physical diseases but also medical practitioners sometimes cause suffering by applying their technical knowledge without regard for the personhood of their patient. Cassel concludes that though "none are more concerned about pain or loss of function than physicians" (ibid., 644), they sometimes cause suffering by seeing a person as divided into a mind, on the one hand, and a body, on the other, and then concluding that the object of their professional concern is only the body. Physicians therefore sometimes cause suffering through "a failure of knowledge and understanding. We lack knowledge, because in working from a dichotomy contrived within a historical context far from our own, we have artificially circumscribed our task in caring for the sick" (ibid.). True empathy focuses on the impact that disease and its treatment have on a patient's ability to lead a meaningful life.

Empathy is a mode of caring. Specifically, it involves caring for the fate or fortune of another human being. Few discussions make it explicit, but empathy is not for those who are flourishing or happy, however easy it is to know how they feel. Empathy is for those who need help or are suffering or struggling in some way. The concept of empathy is relevant to the clinical situation because patients are people in need of help.

1. This idea of professional knowledge as necessarily in the service of some benefit beyond itself is finally Plato's. See Book I of the *Republic*, especially the refutation of Thrasymachus' cynical definition of justice.

The possibility of suffering is the possibility of a degradation of the self by physical disease. Empathy is an understanding of how a disease and its treatment are likely to affect how patients actually live and hope to live their lives. It is to understand, in short, what the disease means to the patient. Only with such understanding do caregivers grasp the basic nature of their role as professional caregivers. The emotion or feeling that some identify with empathy is, in our view, not empathy itself, but a not-uncommon response to empathic understanding. Understanding what a disease means to a patient can certainly result in an emotional response, but empathy is more important than emotion or feeling. It is an understanding based on a reasonably complete knowledge of *who* the patient is, and that provides a general guidance to care and treatment.

Empathic understanding is a basic characteristic of the true clinician and a fundamental requirement for the full development of practical clinical knowledge. Even as the technical demands of clinical practice increase, clinicians who strive for an understanding of the practical, human meaning of disease and treatment can develop their clinical knowledge fully in response to its real purpose. Practitioners and patients alike, after all, are active participants in the clinical exchange. The clinician's task is to adapt clinical knowledge to the care of each new patient. Clinicians who broaden their knowledge in this way can adapt to the specific needs of patients. In this sense, an experienced empathic clinician can note differing responses and techniques. The development of clinical expertise, and its theory, is rooted in such *cumulative*, concrete experience. Empathy, as a comprehension of the meaning of the disease for the patient, is necessary for competence to grown into expertise. Such understanding is not exclusive to nursing but supplies the basis for all expert clinical judgment.

In summary, empathy is not a psychological or emotional experience, nor a psychic leap into the mind of another person, but an openness to, and respect for, the personhood of another. By steering the conception of empathy away from evocative descriptions of a psychological phenomenon, the difficulties with notions of subjectivity and objectivity are obviated. It is no longer a relevant question whether empathy can be objective since it is neither necessary nor possible for the clinician to leave the self behind to experience empathy.

The basis of any helping profession is the welfare of the individual, a sensitivity to people as human beings rather than people as cases. The purpose of both medicine and nursing is to cultivate the welfare of persons and not to simply bring about the successful resolution of cases. In this sense, empathy belongs equally to nurses and doctors, since both physicians and nurses require empathy to develop and exercise expert judgment.

References

American Board of Internal Medicine. 1983. Evaluation of humanistic qualities in the internist. *Annals of Internal Medicine.* 99:720–24.

Bates, B. 1970. Doctor and nurse: Changing roles and relations. *New England Journal of Medicine.* 283:129–34.

Beckman, H., and R. Frankel. 1984. The effect of physician behavior on the collection of data. *Annals of Internal Medicine.* 101:692–96.

Bellet, P., and M. J. Maloney. 1991. The importance of empathy as an interviewing skill in medicine. *Journal of the American Medical Association.* 266:1831–32.

Cassel, E. J. 1982. The nature of suffering and the goals of medicine. *New England Journal of Medicine.* 306:639–45.

Cousins, N. 1985. How patients appraise physicians. *New England Journal of Medicine.* 313:1422–24.

Davis, C. M. 1990. What is empathy, and can empathy be taught? *Physical Therapy.* 70:707–11.

Diers, D. 1990. To profess . . . to be a professional. In *Nursing Trends and Issues,* ed. C. Lindeman and M. McAthie. Springhouse, Penn.: Springhouse.

Ehmann, V. E. 1971. Empathy: Its origin, characteristic, and process. *Perspectives in Psychiatric Care.* 9(2):72–81.

Engle, G. 1977. The need for a new medical model: A challenge for biomedicine. *Science.* 196:129–36.

Gallop, R., W. J. Lancee, and P. E. Garfinkel. 1990. The empathic process and its mediators: A heuristic model. *Journal of Nervous and Mental Disease.* 178:649–54.

Henderson, V. 1960. *The Basic Principles of Nursing Care.* London: International Council of Nurses.

Katz, R. L. 1963. *Empathy: Its Nature and Uses.* New York: Free Press.

Melosh, B. 1982. *The Physician's Hand.* Philadelphia: Temple University Press.

Osler, W. 1904. *Aequanimitas with Other Addresses to Medical Students, Nurses, and Practitioners.* London: Keynes Press.

Rogers, C. 1975. Empathic: An unappreciated way of being. *Counseling Psychologist.* 5(2):2–10.

Stephany, T. 1992. As I see it. *American Nurse.* 24(5):4.

Stillman, P. L., M. Y. Burpeau-DiGregoria, G. Nicholson II, D. L. Sabers, and A. E. Stillman. 1983. Six years of experience using patient instructors to teach interviewing skills. *Journal of Medical Education.* 58:941–46.

Stillman, P. L., M. B. Regan, D. B. Swanson, S. Case, J. McCahan, J. Feinblatt, S. R. Smith, J. Williams, and D. V. Nelson. 1990. An assessment of the clinical skills of fourth-year students at four New England medical schools. *Academic Medicine.* 65:320–25.

Zderad, L. T. 1969. Empathic nursing: Realization of a human capacity. *Nursing Clinics of North America.* 4(4):655–62.

Chapter 9
The Empathic Physician:
Nature and Nurture

SHIMON M. GLICK

Time magazine's cover story on July 31, 1989 (Gibbs 1989, 48), "Doctors and Patients—Image versus Reality," began with a quotation from George Bernard Shaw, "I do not know a single thoughtful and well-informed person who does not feel that the tragedy of illness at present is that it delivers you helplessly into the hands of a profession which you deeply mistrust." *Time*'s following sentence sharpened the criticism with the comment, "That sentiment is mild compared with some of today's reviews."

In an era of almost miraculous advances in every area of medicine, the public's malaise and dissatisfaction relate predominantly to a perceived failure in the physician-patient relationship and not in the sphere of scientific or technologic competence.

There is a growing literature relating to our profession's failure in the caring-empathic dimension, and a substantial portion of it is being written by physicians or their families (Stetten 1981). In *Heartsounds*, Martha Weinman Lear (1980) has written a detailed lament describing the hospitalizations and medical care of her husband, a prominent New York physician, and the lack of communication between physicians and their patients and families even when dealing with medical colleagues. In the paper by the Rabin family (Rabin et al.

1982) the tone is more restrained but the description of physicians' reactions to a colleague's illness is no less sad; here the writers depict the isolation suffered by a distinguished professor of medicine after being stricken with amyotrophic lateral sclerosis.

The literature (Marks and Sachar 1973) also offers a devastating indictment of the administration of narcotics to patients suffering from the pain of cancer or an operation. The resident physicians prescribe inadequate doses of narcotics, the nurses administer only a fraction of the prescribed dose, and the attending senior physicians do not adequately monitor or correct the deficiencies of the junior staff—a depressing indictment of physician behavior—not toward psychoneurotic, geriatric, or similarly "unpopular" patients, but toward the sickest patients, who by any criteria were most deserving, and who should have been expected to receive the very best care. Even more disturbing is the observation that almost a decade after the appearance of this distressing article virtually identical findings were again reported (Angell 1982). The original article, with an accompanying editorial, had not produced the expected change in the behavior of physicians and nurses. A recent poignant description by a British physician (Fenton 1992) of his grandfather's death with inadequate terminal pain relief confirms that we are not dealing with an exclusively North American problem.

It is disturbing indeed that medicine, whose essence is empathy, should stand accused of deficiency in this very quality. It behooves us to examine the possible etiology of such a paradox.

Humanism versus Science and Technology

I reject the commonly held belief that medicine suffers from an inherent conflict between science and technology on the one hand and humanism and empathy on the other hand. Yet a temporal relationship seems to exist between the ascendancy of technology, the advances of science, and the seeming decline in those humanistic qualities of the physician that are so desirable, yet so elusive. If we want to deal effectively with the problem, we must we willing to examine this relationship.

One factor in the apparent decline of compassion is that while science is indeed neutral regarding the human aspects of medicine, the successes of scientific intervention in medicine have served to award it an ever-increasing role in the physician-patient interaction. The unparalleled advances in science and technology have dazzled the medical profession, have virtually monopolized our emphases and education, and have almost inevitably relegated the human aspects of medicine to a secondary role.

A physician sitting day and night by the bedside of a patient with pneumococcal pneumonia does little to cure the patient. But one penicillin injection by a physician who may not know, or even care to know, the patient's name, social status, or emotional state will effect a cure. Is it any wonder then that penicillin, rather than hand holding and empathy, epitomizes modern medicine and that science overshadows compassion?

It is natural also that the fascinating, dramatic, and rapidly advancing fields of scientific medicine will attract and excite the best students and professional minds. The public, too, demand modern, technically sophisticated health care. It is only when this technologically superior care is delivered in a cold and mechanical manner that patients complain.

In the academic world, too, the policy of "publish or perish" naturally emphasizes the discovery of new knowledge. The lay public also awards recognition for such achievement. It is relatively easy to publish an article describing a new enzyme or technique, but more difficult to publish an article on kindness or empathy. Indeed there should be little new in that. Faculty members learn quickly that an hour spent at the laboratory bench can advance them much further during faculty promotional considerations than days spent at a patient's bedside. It would be an unusual faculty promotions committee that would assign major weight to the compassionate qualities of a junior faculty member among the criteria for promotion to professorial rank. Most Western medical systems also provide far greater remuneration for a relatively trivial five-minute technical procedure than for an hour of emotionally wrenching bedside care. Thus, the "carrot and stick" with respect to academic and professional prestige and financial considerations all push in one direction. While society bemoans the qualities of its physicians, the order of priorities favoring technology is a product of society as a whole, and not merely the result of distortion by the medical profession.

A second difficulty resulting from medical advances has been the profession's inevitable fragmentation into subspecialties. The division of a patient between a number of physicians, each concerned with one order or organ-system, makes it difficult for any of the physicians to assume responsibility for the totality of the patient's care. Thus, a frightened patient with a myocardial infarction will be frustrated in spite of his cardiologist's consummate skills in directing a catheter through the twists and turns of his coronary arteries if that physician cannot transcend his narrow focus and also address satisfactorily the patient's overwhelming fears and anxieties. Unfortunately, the selection process that seeks out the superb catheter manipulator does not simultaneously select for compassion and understanding. Nor does the average invasive cardiologist give nearly as much thought and effort toward developing communication skills as toward perfecting manipulative talents.

A third more fundamental problem in the decline of compassion in medicine relates to the physician's motivation. Motivation largely determines the physician's area of interest and approach to patients. The problems of inappropriate motivation are of major magnitude and are not confined to the medical profession but reflect societal trends of the past century. Western educational systems, once based on religious values with emphasis on service to G-d, fellow humans, and society, tended to a certain degree to encourage the development of sensitive, concerned individuals attuned to the needs of their patients.

But our modern Western post-Freudian world now emphasizes happiness and self-fulfillment as the major personal goals. It is not surprising that in a materialistic and permissive environment in which personal satisfaction and actualization are the highest goals, medicine, too, will attract many who want to receive from, rather than give to, the profession. They may be seeking intellectual gratification, prestige, or economic advantage, but often service is not their first priority—neither are the patient's emotional needs.

Most Western medical schools have elaborate medical student selection processes that emphasize scholastic achievement in feeder schools and on entry examinations. The selection process, which favors the brilliant and competitive students, is not geared to discover the empathic sensitive human. Brilliance does not interfere with compassion—the two are essentially unrelated, but if the goal is the production of empathic physicians, conscious efforts must be made in the selection process to identify those candidates who will excel in these areas as well.

The educational process in most medical schools unfortunately perpetuates the initial message, with emphasis on cognitive skills rather than on human qualities. Students may be expelled for failing to accumulate enough factual information or technical skills, but rare indeed is the student whose studies are terminated for a demonstrated lack of empathy. Then there is also the dehumanization and alienation that occurs during the stressful years of medical school. The years of study have been divided by some wags into the precynical and the cynical years, with the blame for this change placed at the feet of the educational establishment. I think these factors have been exaggerated, since the alleged decline in physicians' compassion has coincided paradoxically with a reduction, and not an increase, in work hours and stress. Nevertheless, this student complaint does have some merit and it should not be dismissed cavalierly.

A further aspect of the problem of the empathic physician, not fully appreciated by the public and even by the medical profession itself, is the critical importance of talents and skills. All would agree that motivation and good intentions are insufficient to enable one to perform delicate surgery or to treat complicated metabolic derangements. All the compassion and empathy in the world cannot replace the skills and knowledge of the internist or surgeon. Similarly, all the fine human qualities cannot replace skills in communication, in discerning and diagnosing emotional problems, and in sophisticated management of these difficult and sensitive areas. If physicians are unable to recognize the subtle signs of depression, they can be of little help. If they are frightened of coping with the anxieties of the dying patient because no one taught them how to do so, they may fail, in spite of the best intentions. Most medical schools have heretofore insufficiently stressed the education of physicians in the disciplines and techniques needed to cope with these areas, although there has been a definite improvement of late.

Still another aspect of the education of the physician is its practical rather than theoretical nature. Much teaching takes place at the bedside, and it is what students see there rather than what they hear in the lecture hall that is most likely to influence their ultimate behavior. Students often imitate teachers. Since few of the professors have received training in the field of human interactions, they may not be the appropriate role models. Indeed, most of us attained our status in recognition of our scientific achievements and not because we were devoted and caring physicians. Brilliant laboratory research does not necessarily make a teacher an appropriate model in human relations.

Finally, I would like to focus on an aspect of the physician-patient relationship that epitomizes much of the malaise and dissatisfaction of the physician-patient relationship in modern times. A major cause of tension is the difference between what patients want from their physician and, in contrast, how the physician perceives the encounter. There is major dissonance between the patients' and the physicians' perception. Patients need caring as much as curing. They insist on both. But modern physicians, enthralled with their newly discovered ability to cure, have learned to seek their gratification in this capacity, often forgetting the caring mode and sometimes leaving patients frustrated and angry even when cured. In his classic article, Peabody states, "The reward is to be found in that personal bond which forms the greatest satisfaction of the practice of medicine" (Peabody [1927] 1984, 818). But that message, from an era when medicine could indeed cure very few illnesses, has been eclipsed by the medical miracles of the past few decades and must be resuscitated with much effort and skill.

A Paradigm Integrating Humanism and Science in Medicine

I find useful and essential for the practice of medicine a paradigm that links science and technology inextricably with humanism. Under this scheme

BIOPSYCHOSOCIAL MODEL

↑

UTILIZATION OF *ALL* THE DATA

↑

SCIENTIFIC MEDICINE

↑

IDEAL MEDICAL CARE

↑

COMPASSION

*Figure 1. A paradigm for the integration
of humanism and science in medicine.*

(see Figure 1), it is impossible to provide scientific medicine without humanism, or compassionate medicine without an adequate scientific base.

I start with the fundamental basis of the profession, the essential motivation and driving force of the physician. That basis is *not* science or technology. Neither is it a thirst for knowledge or curiosity, though all these factors and qualities are important. The foundation on which medicine must be based is compassion, that is where it all starts, and without this basis one cannot be a true physician.

If physicians are indeed concerned about the suffering of fellow humans, as if they themselves or members of their own family were ailing, they would want those patients to obtain the most effective care available—ideal medical care— nothing less will do. That ideal care is not homeopathy, nor reflexology, nor whatever alternative medicine is currently in fashion. There is only one legiti- mate school of medicine, and that is scientific medicine. If and when any alter- native form of therapy proves its usefulness by the scientific tools of evidence, it joins mainstream medicine.

It is not enough for physicians to care deeply about patients. That can be done as well or even better by friends, clergy, or social workers. Physicians, if they are to be true to their profession, must act as scientists by examining data, creating hypotheses, and subjecting them to critical scrutiny in an area where controlled scientific observations and proofs are much more difficult than in the laboratory, but there is no alternative.

In carrying out the scientific part of their task, physicians, like any other scientists, must gather *all* the data necessary to reach conclusions. These data may include information from the electron microscope and the computed to- mography scan, but information gleaned from the physical examination and the social history are no less important. In the treatment of pulmonary edema, it is scientifically incompetent to miss a pertinent electrocardiographic finding, but it is no less egregious a *scientific* error to ignore the sodium intake of a derelict, forced by poverty and absent dentures to subsist on canned soups loaded with salt.

The only model that can satisfactorily meet, not just the demands imposed by compassion, but those required by the exactitude of science, is the bio-psychosocial model. A failure of compassion will inevitably lead to *poor science* in medicine because it ignores data critical to the patient's care.

Over the years George Engel has condemned most convincingly the poor science that characterizes the practice of medicine when it ignores the psycho-social dimension. His now classic stories (Engel 1987) of the business executive with the myocardial infarction whose ventricular fibrillation was precipitated by the unsuccessful efforts of the resident physician to obtain arterial blood gases, of the man with massive leg edema who had been sleeping for months in a sitting position in his "home," a cramped Volkswagen auto, are graphic and dramatic. But the hard scientific data supporting his view are no less convincing and continue to accumulate. In patients who have suffered from a myocardial infarction, living alone is no less a risk factor than the classic biochemical or physiological risk factors (Case et al. 1992). The data also clearly show that most physicians repeatedly fail to diagnose overt depression in their patients (Schulberg and Burns 1988; Ormel et al. 1990).

It should therefore be evident that medicine cannot tolerate a dichotomy between its biological and its psychosocial components. The two aspects must exist synergistically if medicine is to offer its full range of benefits to the public.

The Characteristics of the Empathic-Compassionate Physician

Over the years I have developed my own profile for this model physician. I will describe this paragon of virtue and then relate some of the data we have accumulated in a study recently completed at our hospital.

First, compassionate physicians regard human life as unique and of extraordinary importance. They stand in reverent awe of the human being and treat every person with dignity and respect. I have avoided the term *sanctity of life* because of its clearly religious connotations and because the term has been criticized by some leading philosophers (Clouser 1973). But whether sacred or not, a human being should be regarded with a degree of reverence we would not grant to even the most complex or impressive supercomputer or spaceship. I believe that compassion or empathy may weaken unless human life is granted some sort of unique status, both quantitatively and qualitatively, if only for pragmatic reasons.

Second, compassionate physicians have a particular view of their societal role and life goals. They are imbued with values of service to society and of altruism and less with those of self-fulfillment and self-realization. That human beings were placed in the world to serve and not merely to be served was indeed the prevailing view in the Western world for many centuries. It was basically a religious Judeo-Christian view, which in turn represented a major break with that of many prevalent pagan and hedonistic societies, including Greece and Rome. According to such a worldview, human beings exist to serve some higher purpose and not merely to attain their personal needs and goals. Physicians, too, were expected to have chosen their profession as a means of serving humankind. Physicians, along with members of a few selected professions, were considered nobler than their fellow humans, since so much of their energy and activity was socially useful. It was not surprising, then, that the physician was often held in high esteem, as epitomized by Robert Louis Stevenson's remark that the physician was the "flower of civilization."

This view of man's role in society has retreated remarkably in the West coincident with the decline of religion as a major motivating force and the revolutions brought about by Darwin, Freud, and Marx, among others. The decline of this worldview has been accompanied by the overt championing of hedonism, permissiveness, and self-fulfillment as the ultimate goals of life. Ayn Rand's "objectivism" articulated the philosophy of selfishness as an ideal in a most dramatic and focused manner in the novel *The Fountainhead*, in which the hero, an architect, blows up a low-income housing project because the builders deviated from his plans and thereby marred his artistic freedom of expression.

I often have the feeling that the societal pressures in this direction are so overpowering that even individuals who are genuinely committed to the service of others are now often embarrassed to confess to such "outdated" values. The modern narcissistic worldview is problematic for the physician since it clashes head on with altruism and compassion.

As one who is personally committed to religion, I could easily make a good case that the first two qualities mentioned, the belief in the uniqueness of man and of service to a higher goal, may best be classified as representative of a religious world outlook. Such a position—albeit tempting—is true only in part. Compassion can be found among atheists and agnostics and many a nominally religious adherent can be found with poor performance in the interpersonal domain. Yet it is true that the kind of saintly behavior typified by Mother Teresa or Dr. Schweizer is found almost exclusively among those with a deeply religious commitment. What should concern secular societies, which now constitute most of the West, much more is whether or not their ethical distillates, still largely attributable to values inherited from their religious forbears, can continue to be passed on from one generation to the next after they have become uncoupled from their religious moorings. This is one of the major challenges for the ongoing integrity and health of modern Western societies.

Third, compassionate physicians can function best if they are emotionally mature and stable. Irrespective of their philosophy of life, a measure of personal stability and maturity is essential if physicians are to cope adequately with patients' emotional needs and crises.

Here, too, attention must be paid to the environment in which students and physicians function. By its very nature, medical education and subsequent practice is physically and emotionally taxing. Rigorous and stressful training is unavoidable if only to weed out unsuitable individuals at an early stage. But callous and inconsiderate treatment of students and residents during times of personal difficulties (Silver and Glicken 1990; Sheehan et al. 1990) must, inevitably, take its toll and may result in undesirable and impaired behavior toward patients. The environment in which physicians work must reinforce empathy. This is possible even in stressful surroundings if a conscious effort is made. All too often the stress and pressures intrinsic to medicine are used to rationalize inappropriate behavior on the part of the physician.

The fourth essential for the empathic physician is skill in the art of medicine. Sobbing uncontrollably along with a distressed patient may represent the ultimate in empathy. But the patient needs effective empathy. In order to accomplish this end, one needs training in both diagnostic and therapeutic skills. While it is difficult to alter basic attitudes and character traits, the skills can and must be taught. Many physicians still believe that such skills are acquired spontaneously by experience, but in spite of years of medical practice many physicians never feel comfortable handling psychosocial problems. Much of the reticence and hesitation on the part of physicians to deal with the emotional component of patients' illnesses is due to their general feeling of inadequacy and incompetence in this domain. Most of us enjoy doing what we do well and avoid areas in which we feel less competent. During recent years, increasing numbers of medical schools have begun formal instruction in interpersonal communication skills, often both to teachers and to students, with impressive results.

Finally, compassionate physicians possess a hypertrophied conscience and strive constantly for ethical excellence. They examine and re-examine their performance to compare it with a preconceived ideal.

My colleagues and I have recently completed a study in our hospital which attempted to characterize the personal, social, and organizational factors contributing to the creation and sustenance of the "empathic compassionate" (e-c) physicians, as defined by their peers. We distributed a questionnaire to 324 full-time physicians at our 750-bed major teaching hospital and asked them each to identify in rank order the five resident physicians and the five attending physicians who in their opinion fitted the provided description of the e-c physician. We received 231 completed questionnaires (71.3 percent response). We then ranked the hospital's physicians according to the number of times they were cited by colleagues. Those who were cited by at least 10 colleagues (27 attending physicians, 19 resident physicians) were classified as e-c physicians. We then identified two control groups, one which included physicians with no citations and an intermediate group with few citations.

In phase two of the project we distributed detailed questionnaires (270 questions) to 308 physicians and received full responses from 214 (69.5 percent response). The questionnaire evaluated by a variety of standard test measures self-esteem, anxiety, social attitudes, empathy, degree of consultation with other professionals, work attitudes, socialization, home background, role models, motivation in selecting specialty, work habits, attitudes toward place of work, work satisfaction, and burnout.

We found that the e-c physicians tended to be younger, Israeli educated, had a higher degree of self-confidence and a low level of anxiety. They had more universalistic and less stereotyped attitudes toward patients and were more conscious of psychosocial factors. In characterizing a "good physician" they tended to emphasize devotion, willingness to assume responsibility and to invest much time and effort in their profession, and placed significantly less emphasis on status, monetary reward, personal appearance, and self-confidence. In selecting a specialty, the e-c physician gave less emphasis to the prestige of the specialty, life-style, patient mix, earnings, and research. The e-c physicians tended to consult other physicians more frequently and were less offended by patient requests for such consultation. They reported longer working hours in teaching and study at the hospital and less time on moonlighting outside the hospital to supplement earnings. E-c physicians, more frequently than others, reported a dominant maternal influence on their behavior. Among ideologies influencing their behavior the e-c group had a higher proportion with religion as a dominant influence than did other groups. The e-c physicians were more pleased with their relations with colleagues and had more confidence in the system and in their ability to influence it. But they were more dissatisfied than the others with their lack of time for work and for family.

In spite of the fairly extensive nature of this study, it nevertheless has many limitations, aside from its geographic and cultural bias. It is based purely on peer ratings, and its results are dependent on the validity of each of the measurement tools used. But to a major extent, I was personally pleased in that several of my observational hypotheses found some support.

The physician with the desirable qualities seems to be motivated more by altruism and less by selfish life goals; there is a tendency for religious influence to be stronger; e-c physicians seem more secure and less anxious in their relationships with their peers and their patients, and they are more conscientious and demanding of themselves. Several of the associated characteristics that were identified make it seem likely that e-c physicians would be rated higher by their colleagues in overall competence. This assessment is likely because they spent more hours in teaching and study and were more willing to consult with colleagues, had better motivations for the practice of medicine, and were more at peace with themselves in the profession and with their work environment. The likelihood that e-c physicians excel in other professional qualities besides compassion and empathy belies the alleged inherent contradiction between the scientific and the humanistic types of physicians.

Creating the Empathic Physician

Clearly the task of creating the empathic physician does not begin in medical school. By the time most medical students embark on their studies, their basic attitudes and inclinations reflect the first two formative decades of their lives. Therefore one of the critical tasks of medical schools, if they are interested in promoting empathy in their final product, is the appropriate selection of students from among the many candidates who apply. Although there is no foolproof method for predicting subsequent empathic behavior in a candidate at the time of application to medical school, it seems likely that, through a conscious effort by the admissions committee, one can obtain a pool of students with more empathic tendencies than by chance alone or by relying on purely academic achievement.

Medical schools rely heavily on personal interviews; every successful candidate is interviewed by two pairs of interviewers for about forty-five minutes each (Antonovsky 1987). During these semi-structured interviews, specific evidence of empathic behavior in the candidate's past record is sought, and penetrating questions are often asked to elicit attitudes in the areas under concern. To illustrate, a candidate who has spent a year of her life volunteering to work with families bereaved by war (a true example) is more likely to demonstrate subsequent empathic behavior than one whose previous activities have all been totally self-centered. We are now in the process of seeking some objective tests to compare students selected this way to those selected from the same pool of applicants at other Israeli medical schools. It has previously been shown that the students selected by our interview process score higher on the Rest Ethical Defining Test (Benor et al. 1984). Many anecdotes from faculty members who

have taught at other medical schools in Israel report a distinct difference between our students and those at the other schools in their attitudes toward
patients. Our own data reported earlier in this paper and those of Linn (Linn
1987), who described several sociodemographic and premedical school factors
which correlate with physicians' humanistic performance, suggest that with
more extensive research we may be able to provide better candidate profiles of
students who are more likely to be empathic.

I believe that one can obtain general agreement that the best way to produce
empathic, caring physicians would be for all role models interacting with the
students to be empathic, compassionate individuals. If Francis Peabody were the
teacher attending on each ward round during undergraduate and graduate
training, this book would probably be superfluous. In the book describing Case
Western Reserve University's bold experiment in medical education (Williams
1980), Williams points out that the major influence on Dean Wearn, the architect of their revolution in medical education, was Francis Peabody. Peabody's
classic article "The Care of the Patient" has been quoted continuously and
reprinted frequently for more than sixty years, because in Williams's words "it
has been too seldom heeded in the modern age of science and technology."
Peabodys are few and far between and seem to be growing rarer. Therefore
conscious efforts must be made in the educational system to heighten the student's sensitivities to the sick and suffering human being.

In describing what we do at the Ben Gurion University Faculty of Health
Sciences it is often difficult to decide which of the specific facets of our program
accomplishes what. So many components interact simultaneously.

A unique feature of our program, which may seem only ritually symbolic, is
the administration of the physician's oath to the *entering* class at the graduation
ceremony of the senior class. This step is intended to impress on the incoming
young men and women that even as students they already have an obligation to
serve and not just to be served by the patients they will examine. The timing of
the oath at a more impressionable stage in the physician's training than at the
end of medical school may have some impact.

During a several-week preschool summer program, our students begin to
learn basic communication skills, have discussions on issues of medical ethics,
and are taken to visit underprivileged communities in the region in order to
begin to appreciate parts of society to which many of the students have never
been exposed. During the first two years (of a six-year program), which in Israel
traditionally covers just basic sciences, the students have extensive clinical exposure. During the first year, four full weeks and one day of every other week are
devoted to clinical studies. A major portion of the time is devoted to communication skills. The student is exposed to the worlds of their patients and their

families. Unlike such exposure during clinical years, when the student is appropriately preoccupied, stressed, and often overwhelmed by learning pathophysiology, physical diagnosis, and therapeutics simultaneously, the first-year student has little alternative but to focus almost exclusively on the patient's personal problems. These clinical sessions take place in several settings: on a general medical ward, in a maternal and child health station, in a geriatric setting, and in a community clinic.

In one clinical week, students follow the hospitalization procedure of a single patient from the emergency room through discharge, sharing the *experience* (Carmel and Bernstein 1986). Some students are also "hospitalized" and subsequent discussions with classmates elaborate on their reactions to the process. For the past two years we have introduced a new locale: that of the disabled patient. In this setting the students meet with the blind, the deaf, and the mentally retarded and learn of their problems and of the way they interact with other people. Students emerge emotionally moved from this experience, and from our feedback sessions it is clear that empathy has been significantly enhanced.

In the second year there are clinical weeks dealing with cancer, including interviews with dying patients and surviving families, in addition to basic science and the clinical aspects of cancer. The students also have a week devoted to families in crisis, which focuses on patients admitted to intensive care units and the impact on them and their families.

By the end of the first two years of medical school, students have acquired a profound appreciation of what it is like to be ill, the impact on the psyche and the family, the differing cultural reactions to illness, and the empathic way of dealing with patients and their families during a variety of crises at home, in the hospital, in the community, and in the workplace.

In his recent provocative paper, Spiro makes a simple but most profound comment: "Conversation helps to develop empathy" (Spiro 1992, 844). The frenetic pace on today's medical wards discourages the resident physicians from taking time to converse with patients (Rabkin 1982; Glick 1988). These physicians are harried and distressed themselves from running from emergency to emergency. Anything less than a life or death situation seems of trivial importance relative to the series of crises in which they are constantly involved. To expect medical students during their medical clerkships to learn empathy in that environment from their fatigued mentors is unreasonable—and indeed they do not. It is for this reason that I feel that early clinical exposure is of such critical importance. I am convinced that meeting patients first in a context which emphasizes the psychosocial aspects of medicine rather than the biomedical facets has the effect of "imprinting" a certain attitude and behavior pattern. The subsequent erosion that inevitably occurs when the students work with the usual resident and attending physicians, only a small minority of whom are Peabodys, fails to eliminate completely the deep impact of the many conversations with patients and families during the students' most impressionable phase.

During the clinical years the students spend required clerkships in family medicine and ambulatory care pediatrics where the psychosocial aspects of medicine receive considerable emphasis. Unfortunately most of our hospital-based clerkships have little planned formal teaching in these areas. We are a very small faculty and those individuals with the requisite skills and interest are already overly committed to teaching duties beyond their ability. We have been impressed with the recently published program of Almy's group (Almy et al. 1992) that focuses on the application of the social sciences and the humanities. This takes place in the final year of medical school and is patient-centered and problem-based.

In the final year there is a course of several weeks, "The Physician and Society." This multidisciplinary course focuses on medical ethics, legal medicine, medical anthropology, medical economics, and on the social relationship of psychiatry in society. The course is a kind of final summary of some of the broader issues in the interaction of the modern socially conscious physician with society.

Another aspect of our medical school is the involvement of the student as an active partner in curriculum planning and evaluation. The students are consulted concerning many aspects of the school's operation, and senior students are involved as teaching assistants for junior classes. This interaction minimizes alienation, gives the students a feeling that they are members of an important health team and not merely the passive recipients of factual knowledge. The students are also taught to assume the role of agents of change not just with respect to the school but with respect to the community problems they encounter. The students are taught that they share responsibility for what is wrong and that they have a duty to attempt to effect change. We believe that a medical school atmosphere in which students are treated with respect and dignity enhances the students' empathic behavior.

Our students have had a positive impact on the behavior of their clinical teachers, raising issues that are often ignored by their mentors and thereby heightening the sensitivity of even relatively callous and cynical senior physicians. A good number of our graduates have now begun to take their places on our faculty, thus reinforcing the positive attitude that we seek in our students.

Internship supervisors throughout Israel have repeatedly favorably evaluated the behavior and skills of our graduates in the humanistic interpersonal domain. In addition, dozens of anecdotal reports from patients, both hospitalized and in the community, have noted that Beer-Sheva graduates behave significantly more empathically than graduates of the other medical schools they have encountered.

A research project is currently underway, conducted as a part of a doctoral thesis in sociology at another Israeli university, that will observe physicians' empathic behavior in the field in an attempt to determine specifically whether observable differences exist between graduates of the different schools in Israel.

I have provided just a few examples of programs that we think may enhance the development of empathy in physicians. I am confident that there are other equally effective or better programs to achieve these goals. Clearly much more needs to be learned in this area and certainly more needs to be done. It is encouraging to see an apparent upsurge of interest in this field as evidenced by this book and by the literature cited herein. Yet even today with the increased attention devoted to the behavioral sciences, a recent most disconcerting figure cited by the Robert Wood Johnson Foundation Commission on Medical Education (Haggerty et al. 1992, 74–78) shows that out of a total of 72,000 positions in all the American medical schools, there are only 126 budgeted faculty positions in the behavioral sciences. These figures contrast with 1,902 positions in biochemistry, 1,871 positions in physiology, and 2,553 in cell biology, genetics, and microbiology. Clearly there is much room for improvement.

The relative neglect of the behavioral aspects of medicine exemplifies an unfortunate aspect of our modern professional and academic life. Plato is quoted as saying, "An unexamined life is one not worth living." True professionals, in whatever field, are forever striving to upgrade their performance. Surgeons will not be satisfied until they have perfected their operative techniques, cardiologists until they can diagnose the most complex arrhythmia. In an academic environment, we have set up a variety of mechanisms for peer evaluation and for self-evaluation—mortality conferences, clinical pathological conferences, chart reviews, statistics—the key word is *accountability*. In our personal lives, too, most of us in the professional and academic world have honed and refined our esthetic tastes and our technological demands. We seek high-fidelity record players with sound refinements beyond our ear's ability to detect, gourmet foods and quality wines whose "desired" bouquets are often beyond our capacity to identify on double-blind tests. Even those who never manage to arrive on time insist on watches that are accurate to the millisecond. The standards of performance demanded by us in many areas of endeavor far outstrip our legitimate "needs." Yet, continual striving for improvement and excellence seems almost inherent in the physician's makeup and has much to commend it.

But what do we modernists do to similarly upgrade our ethical behavior, our compassion, our humanism? How often do we review our interpersonal behavior in the same critical manner that we review a difficult medical case? Was the proper word or phrase used with the patient, the student, the colleague at the appropriate time? Do we strive for excellence in these spheres as well? These sensitive matters are generally taken for granted, they are apparently regarded either as elementary or as relatively unimportant. But they are neither simple nor trivial.

Basically, the modern world in which we live has set for itself an order of priorities that does not demand meticulous examination of behavior by a rigorous, ethical standard. Unless we, as educators, do impose ethical demands on behavior, we cannot expect to demonstrate the level of excellence in the interpersonal sphere in those areas that we do stress.

In this context, I would like to describe a facet of the character of that unusual intellectual and scholar, Benjamin Franklin, as an example of what was socially and intellectually acceptable in an era. His example should highlight the failings of our modern world and shed some light on fundamental causes of problems such as lack of empathy.

In his autobiography, Benjamin Franklin wrote (Franklin 1950, 101), "It was about this time I conceived the bold and arduous project of arriving at moral perfection." He described his initial difficulties with his task, and then, with his characteristic systematism, he decided upon a list of thirteen virtues that he deemed important. These were temperance, silence, order, resolution, frugality, industry, sincerity, justice, moderation, cleanliness, tranquility, chastity, and humility. He kept a daily performance record for each of these values in a little notebook. He concluded, "On the whole, though I never arrived at the perfection I had been so ambitious of obtaining, but fell short of it, yet I was, by the endeavor, a better and a happier man than I otherwise should have been if I had not attempted it." I am sufficiently in touch with reality to realize that this utopian model of self-examination is not one that is likely to be implemented by most modern medical students and physicians. But this conceptual model does have a message for us. Just as the virtuosic violinist, surgeon, or athlete trains, reviews, and practices for the artistic, technical, or physical performance, so there is room for similar review of one's interpersonal behavior. If we are to place empathy in its rightful place in our profession's order of priorities, we should devote sufficient time and effort to that endeavor, just as to any area in which we strive to excel. Empathy is too important to be left to the medical school's specialists in the behavioral sciences. Certainly these qualities should not be the exclusive province of the alternative medical practitioners of "holistic" medicine who are endeavoring with some success to fill the vacuum we have created. These attributes must become the concern of the most highly skilled physicians and the outstanding teachers who strive for perfection in every other area of endeavor. We must teach and demonstrate by our actions that technically outstanding patient care lacking in compassion is no less a failure than an empathic but scientifically disastrous effort.

In summary, I suggest that the creation of empathic physicians requires *conscious* attention to ethical excellence and compassion if we are to succeed in educating a generation of physicians who can live up to the rich tradition of the profession and who can simultaneously care for, as well as cure, the malaise of both physicians and patients.

References

Almy, T. P., K. K. Colby, M. Zubkoff, et al. 1992. Health, society and the physician: Problem-based learning of the social sciences and humanities: Eight years of experience. *Annals of Internal Medicine.* 116:569–74.

Angell, M. 1982. The quality of mercy (Editorial). *New England Journal of Medicine.* 306:98–99.

Antonovsky, A. 1987. Medical student selection at the Ben-Gurion University of the Negev. *Israel Journal of Medical Sciences* 23:969–75.

Benor, D. E., N. Notzer, T. J. Sheehan, and G. R. Norman. 1984. Moral reasoning as a criterion for admission to medical school. *Medical Education.* 18:423–28.

Carmel, S., and J. Bernstein. 1986. Identifying with the patient: An intensive programme for medical students. *Medical Education.* 20:432–36.

Carmel, S., and S. M. Glick. Unpublished data.

Case, R. B., A. J. Moss, N. Case, M. McDermott, and S. Eberly. 1992. Living alone after myocardial infarction: Impact on prognosis. *Journal of the American Medical Association.* 267:515–19.

Clouser, D. 1973. The sanctity of life: An analysis of a concept. *Annals of Internal Medicine.* 78:119–25.

Engel, G. L. 1987. Physician-scientists and scientific physicians: Resolving the humanism-science dichotomy. *American Journal of Medicine.* 82:107–11.

Fenton, A. 1992. The ultimate failure. *British Medical Journal.* 305:1027.

Franklin, B. 1950 ed. *The Autobiography of Benjamin Franklin and Selections from His Other Writings.* Edited by H. S. Commager. New York: Modern Library.

Gibbs, N. 1989. Sick and tired. *Time.* 134:48.

Glick, S. M. 1988. The impending crises in internal medicine training programs. *American Journal of Medicine.* 84:929–32.

Haggerty, R. J., S. W. Bloom, D. Mechanic, and H. Pardes. 1992. *Report of the Commission's Subcommittee on the Behavioral Sciences in Medical Education in Transition (Robert Wood Johnson Foundation Commission on Medical Education): The Sciences of Medical Practice.* Princeton, N.J.: Robert Wood Johnson Foundation.

Lear, M. W. 1980. *Heartsounds.* New York: Simon and Schuster.

Linn, L. S. 1987. Sociodemographic and premedical school factors related to postgraduate physicians' humanistic performance. *Western Journal of Medicine.* 147:99–103.

Marks, R. M., and E. J. Sachar. 1973. Undertreatment of medical inpatients with narcotic analgesics. *Annals of Internal Medicine.* 78:173–81.

Ormel, J., W. Vanden Brink, M. W. J. Koeter, et al. 1990. Recognition, management and outcome of psychological disorders in primary care: A naturalistic follow-up study. *Psychological Medicine.* 20:909–23.

Peabody, F. W. [1927] 1984. The care of the patient. *Journal of the American Medical Association.* [88:877–82] 252:813–18.

Rabin, D., P. L. Rabin, and R. Rabin. 1982. Compounding the ordeal of ALS—Isolation from my fellow physicians. *New England Journal of Medicine.* 307:506–9.

Rabkin, M. 1982. The SAG index. *New England Journal of Medicine.* 307:1350–51.

Schulberg, H. C., and B. J. Burns. 1988. Mental disorders in primary care: Epidemiologic, diagnostic, and treatment research directions. *General Hospital Psychology.* 10:79–87.

Sheehan, K. H., D. V. Sheehan, K. White, A. Leibowitz, and D. C. Baldwin, Jr. 1990. A pilot study of medical student "abuse": Student perceptions of mistreatment and misconduct in medical school. *Journal of the American Medical Association.* 263:533–37.

Silver, H. K., and A. D. Glicken. 1990. Medical student abuse: Incidence, severity and significance. *Journal of the American Medical Association.* 263:527–32.

Spiro, H. 1992. What is empathy and can it be taught? *Annals of Internal Medicine.* 116:843–46.

Stetten, D., Jr. 1981. Coping with blindness. *New England Journal of Medicine.* 305:458–60.

Williams, G. 1980. *Western Reserve's Experiment in Medical Education and Its Outcome.* New York: Oxford University Press.

Chapter 10
. . . And the Least of These
Is Empathy

RICHARD L. LANDAU

It is essential to start with definitions. In the minds of some people, empathy and sympathy are almost interchangeable terms. They are not! According to the *Random House Unabridged Dictionary of the English Language* "empathy is the intellectual identification with or vicarious experiencing of the feelings, thoughts, or attitudes of another" and "sympathy is the fact or power of sharing the feelings of another, especially in sorrow or trouble; fellow feeling, compassion or commiseration." The distinction is crucial to the positions taken here. One can be sympathetic and understanding and commiserate with another person without placing oneself in the same position.

In May of 1992, Howard Spiro published "What Is Empathy and Can It Be Taught?" in the *Annals of Internal Medicine* (Spiro 1992). In this article he extols the virtue and usefulness of invoking empathy in the practice of medicine. In making his case, Spiro comes perilously close to expressing an antiscientific approach for the future of medicine. To avoid the charge that I have misinterpreted him, let me quote:

The author gratefully acknowledges the constructive suggestions of Clifford W. Gurney and Theodore N. Pullman.

The increased emphasis on molecular biology to the exclusion of the humanities encourages students to focus not on patients, but on diseases. A desk, Nagel reminds us, is more than its spaces and electrons (Nagel 1961). In the 21st century as technology triumphs, empathy will need more attention than equanimity . . . science was once a puny force that had little attraction for those wishing to care for the sick. In the 20th century, however, much has been learned. The advantages in science have been so transfixing and the acceleration of knowledge has grown so compelling that Nagel's desk has lost its solidity. Physicians need to relearn the body, and empathy can help us regain our feeling.

To Spiro, when science triumphs, the humanities are the losers. He not only invokes a struggle of which many of us were unaware, but proposes that empathy will balance the contest.

In disagreeing with him, I shall first point out that rather than excluding the humanities from medical practice and education, the scientific advances of the past quarter century have brought with them an increased awareness of humanistic concerns by the profession. It is also not clear from Spiro's presentation that deficiencies in humanistic concerns, if they exist, would be corrected if physicians were deliberately more empathic. Moreover, he has failed to consider any possible negative effects of more empathic physician-patient relations.

The rapid advances of scientific medicine with the introduction of truly spectacular life-extending technologies have led inevitably to ethical considerations never foreseen by practitioners during the first half of this century. Then the ethos of physicians—doing what they could to comfort and heal for all patients without discrimination—was uncomplicated and sufficient. But the availability of a novel life-extending technology (dialysis for renal failure), originally in very limited supply, brought forth the consideration of which individuals with the qualifying disease should be selected for treatment. These soul-searing decisions were, I believe, the first ones in which disinterested lay people represented the public in helping physicians make the difficult selections (Scribner 1964). From this introduction, the appointment of ethics committees with public and professional members spread rapidly to advise in the growing number of difficult medical decisions and in clinical research programs. Thus by 1982 Steven Toulmin could write his perceptive article entitled "How Medicine Saved the Life of Ethics" (Toulmin 1982).

Quite properly some physicians saw the need to move from ad hoc ethical decision making to a more scholarly approach to medical ethics. More important, the widespread medical and public health education of the public brought nonmedical academic ethicists into the field. Through their professional associations, articles, and books, ethical aspects of the humanities have permeated medical education and practice. Courses on medical ethics have been added to curricula and invited lectures on the subject have become a commonplace for house staffs and practicing physicians. It is difficult to say in 1993 that appropriate ethical concerns have not been woven into medical education and practice.

In addition, some deans and other medical educators have included humanistic educational offerings, in addition to ethics, in response to complaints that physicians had become so imbued with the technical aspects of medical care that they were neglecting the personal or humanistic aspects. The evidence for such a change in the attitude of physicians or medical students is largely hearsay. It is another example of the saying that if an accusation is made with sufficient frequency, it takes on the aura of fact. Some physicians in all generations have always been criticized for not caring. Novelists, playwrights, artists, and cartoonists have depicted the idealistic, sensitive, and caring physicians as well as their cold, cynical, laboratory-oriented or money-grubbing contemporaries. The scientific basis of medicine was blamed for some of the public attitude many years before anyone ever dreamed of molecular biology—the present bugaboo according to Spiro. For those critics of medicine who believe that the exciting advances in molecular biology and medicine have a special facility for warping the character and caring attitudes of physicians, George Bernard Shaw's preface to *The Doctors' Dilemma* (Shaw cited in Landau 1989) written in the first decade of this century should be compulsory reading. His caustic wit emphasized the physicians' grasping for money and prestige over utilizing science, some of which was not good, and caring little for anything but their own welfare.

Physicians' attitudes toward using advanced scientific technology must be examined in the context of the society in which they live and work. The practice of medicine is no longer looked upon with the mystical air that it possessed as recently as the 1940s—an era that I have personally experienced. Americans in all walks of life are now remarkably aware of diseases, therapies, and diagnostic modalities. They seem to be hungry for every new grain of medical information provided by the media. They often hear about published advances in medicine before the physicians' journal is delivered. So, like Marshall Field's successful motto, "Give the lady what she wants" (Wendt and Kogan 1952), the physician who offers effective scientifically based treatment and advanced diagnostic procedures is usually being sensitive to the patient's desires. It is what the educated public, eager for medical knowledge, has learned to expect. It is thus humane for physicians (presumably with sound judgment) to make all the products of scientific advance available to all patients. Sometimes the physician must even be extravagant in ordering special procedures in order to satisfy or reassure the patient and family. This is, incidentally, one of the reasons it will be difficult to curb the rising cost of medical care.

The idea that physicians should be cultivated and broadly educated in the humanities and social sciences is certainly not an original concept. William Osler, probably the most influential medical leader and educator of this century, was dedicated to this view and did much to advance it (Osler 1932). He read voraciously and encouraged all physicians to do the same. His minimum recommendation: thirty minutes every night before retiring. Any deficiencies in the social and humanistic education of today's physicians can properly be ascribed to their secondary school and premedical college education. The premedical students' course selection is usually dominated by the science courses they like or believe will help them gain admission to medical school. This is just one facet of the failure of American colleges and universities to assure that their graduates have a liberal education. College faculties have also defaulted on this obligation for students majoring in the humanities and social sciences. These students often graduate deplorably ignorant in the natural sciences and thus, despite an interest in medical concerns, are fearful and suspicious of what scientific advances may offer for medicine and society. For this reason, they sometimes find it difficult to acquire a comfortable and trusting relationship with physicians. It has been much easier for the college faculties to offer a multitude of electives than to define the liberal education and provide it. If medical school faculties believe that beginning students are ill-prepared in the humanities (and some certainly are), they need only modify requirements for admission. To attempt to make up for this deficiency during the already crowded medical curriculum is mere game playing.

Osler also bears a major responsibility for including the essential biological sciences in the education and the practice of American physicians. His message as a pioneering professor as well as in his speeches and essays was that knowledge of the biological sciences needed to be amalgamated with the cultural attributes he considered essential for members of this profession. His insistence on preserving the scientific method is clear from his frequent reminders on note taking. He regarded detached equanimity in patient management as an essential attribute to be cultivated.

> No quality takes rank with imperturbability. . . . Imperturbability means coolness and presence of mind under all circumstances, calmness amid storm, clearness of judgment in moments of grave peril, immobility, impassiveness . . . the physician who has the misfortune to be without it, who betrays indecision and worry and who shows that he is flustered . . . rapidly loses the confidence of his patients. . . . Cultivate then, gentlemen, such a judicious measure of obtuseness as will enable you to meet the exigencies of practice with firmness and cour-

age, without, at the same time, hardening the human heart by which we live (Osler 1932, 3–4).

Francis Peabody is the other physician who has had an immense positive influence on medical education and the quality of medical care in this country. His lecture "The Care of the Patient" appeared in the *Journal of the American Medical Association* in 1927 (Peabody [1927] 1984). Almost at the start he said, "The most common criticism made at present by older practitioners is that young graduates have been taught a great deal about the mechanism of disease, but very little about the practice of medicine—or, to put it more bluntly, they are too scientific." In disagreeing, Peabody then went on to say that "[the practice of medicine] is an art, based to an increasing extent on the medical sciences, but comprising much that still remains outside the realm of any science. The art of medicine and the science of medicine are not antagonistic but supplementary to each other." He then provided an eloquent description of the blending of medical science with the sympathetic understanding of the life of patients, whether the disease be organic or functional. He emphasized that getting to know the patient should be regarded as a major portion of the art of medicine. He explained how the information thus obtained about the patient's symptoms, pattern of living, family life, and so forth should be integrated with the physical aspects, including test results and special examinations, the total comprising the *scientific* evaluation of the patient's problems. This paper was reprinted in 1984 as a "landmark" contribution in celebration of the one hundred years of the *Journal of the American Medical Association* (Peabody [1927] 1984). The commentary accompanying the reprinting, written by David Rabin and his wife, Pauline, was almost equally prescient (Rabin and Rabin 1984). It is of more than passing interest that both Peabody and the Rabins knew that they were terminally ill when they wrote their articles.

So what of empathy? The word does not appear in the Peabody or Rabin essays. Nor could I find it in the eight articles by Osler that I read. It is a fair guess, however, that Osler is frowning on the idea of its enthusiastic incorporation into medical practice, given his position favoring scientific imperturbability. The aphorism "A physician who cares for himself has a fool for a physician" has been credited to Osler (Bean 1961).

I believe that Howard Spiro would agree that today's medical curriculum orients the student toward an objective, dispassionate view of the patient and his illness. Anatomy, as the introductory course, is important in this regard, because it brings the student face to face with death from the start. It is the beginning of a desensitizing considered essential for the future physician. Alan Gregg described this process more dramatically. "It is commonly known that medical students dissect the bodies of the dead; it is less commonly realized that these same dead do a good deal of cutting, probing and pulling at the minds of their youthful dissectors. What most of us sought that first day among the naked, stark dead in the dissecting room was detachment—detachment enough to stand and view the machinery devoid of spirit, detachment and time enough to compose life with stinking death" (Gregg 1957, 25). In the context of Gregg's essay, such desensitization could well be termed the deempathization required to enable the physician to make sound, scientifically based medical decisions. As the students progress from normal human biology and physiology to pathology and then intimate and responsible contact with patients, it is not unusual for them to be disturbed and to personalize one disorder or another. Additional desensitization or deempathization becomes essential in order to face and care for sick patients without alarming them. This is accomplished by multiplying the students' encounters with patients and by gradually increasing their responsibility. The scientific diagnosis of the patient requires the objective evaluation and integration of all available information. Sound therapeutic decisions necessitate the detached assessment of the diagnosis with consideration of all facets of the patient's life situation. It is not easy to find a place for empathy in this scenario.

Excellent physicians are those who spend time with the patient and thereby gain an understanding of both the clinical problem and the patient's life situation. They must be sensitive, appreciating nuances that creep into the patient's conversation, and sympathetic without always allowing the patient to know it. The patient regards the physician as an authority and wants the opinions and the decisions of a scholarly, experienced expert. Physicians who deliberately cultivate empathy, who place themselves in the patient's position, will not be able to reliably fulfill all of these requirements. For example, physicians who are empathic may be so emotionally involved with their patients (Spiro speaks of passion as a desired result of empathy) that their body language and verbal hesitancy may contradict what they are saying. More important, by placing themselves in their patients' position, they may be unable to make the best decision. In short, encouraging physicians to cultivate empathy in their relations with patients will undermine their ability to function as wise, understanding doctors who give of themselves in guiding patients through life's concerns and illnesses. Indeed it has been suggested that physicians in our largely secular society have—usually without appreciating it—functioned as generic priests, the persons to whom many go with their problems and troubles (Landau and Gustafson 1984).

There are obvious situations in which empathy is almost inevitable. If physicians have experienced the same disease or symptoms as a patient, placing themselves in that patient's position may become almost automatic. Having experienced the disorder will almost certainly assist in making the diagnosis and appreciating the patient's pain and discomfort. Whenever the physician is empathic, however, wisdom dictates that every effort should be made to minimize the emotion when making decisions and speaking to the patient. Fortunately there are a number of circumstances in which empathy is virtually impossible: in pediatrics, a heterosexual dealing with a homosexual, a woman physician dealing with male sexual drive, a man caring for a woman in labor or at menopause.

Effective physicians give patients sufficient time to react and ask questions and learn that they have a sense of humor. They will be sensitive, sympathetic, imperturbable, understanding, and occasionally empathic, but by far the least employed of these traits will be empathy.

References

Bean, William B., ed. 1961. *Sir William Osler: Aphorisms from His Bedside Teachings and Writings*. Springfield: Chas. C. Thomas.

Gregg, A. 1957. *For Future Doctors*. Chicago: University of Chicago Press.

Landau, R. L., and J. M. Gustafson. 1984. Death is not the enemy. *Journal of the American Medical Association*. 252:2458.

Landau, W. M. 1989. The doctor's dilemma: Problems that do not go away. *Perspectives in Biology and Medicine*. 32:505–12.

Nagel, E. 1961. *The Structure of Science: Problems in the Logic of Scientific Explanation*. New York: Harcourt Brace & World.

Osler, W. 1932. *Aequanimitas with Other Addresses to Medical Students, Nurses, and Practitioners of Medicine*. 3d ed. Philadelphia: Blakiston.

Peabody, F. W. [1927] 1984. The care of the patient. *Journal of the American Medical Association*. [88:877–82] 252:813–18.

Rabin, P. R., and D. Rabin. 1984. The care of the patient: Francis Peabody revisited. *Journal of the American Medical Association*. 252:819–20.

Scribner, B. H. 1964. Ethical problems of using artificial organs to sustain life. *American Society of Artificial Internal Organs, Transactions*. 10:209–12.

Spiro, H. 1992. What is empathy and can it be taught? *Annals of Internal Medicine*. 116:843–46.

Toulmin, S. 1982. How medicine saved the life of ethics. *Perspectives in Biology and Medicine*. 32:72–79.

Wendt, L., and H. Kogan. 1952. *Give the Lady What She Wants*. Chicago: Rand McNally.

Chapter 11
Selective Empathy

RICHARD E. PESCHEL
AND ENID PESCHEL

Empathy: The intellectual identification with or vicarious experiencing of the feelings, thoughts, or attitudes of another.

Empathy can be a powerful and extremely useful tool for a physician. One can argue that physicians and other health professionals who develop empathic relationships with their patients make better healers because they have a more compassionate understanding of their patients. One might claim that empathy may be the single most distinguishing characteristic of the superior physician. American medicine is built on the foundations of scientific knowledge and the scientific method,.however. This scientific underpinning of American medicine introduces both restrictions and responsibilities for the empathic physician.

Empathy in the Context of Current Scientific Knowledge

Art can crystallize and focus our attention on many experiences in life, and opera has eloquently portrayed many aspects of the doctor-patient relationship. There is perhaps no greater representation of the empathic physician than Dr. Grenvil in Giuseppe Verdi's masterpiece, *La Traviata*, which made its

110

debut in 1853. Set in the mid-nineteenth century, the opera centers on the stormy love affair between a young courtesan, Violetta, and a young man from a respectable provincial family, Alfredo. Even though Violetta is stricken with consumption and realizes that she may soon die of her disease, she makes the supreme sacrifice of giving up her beloved Alfredo for the sake of Alfredo's sister and his father.

Lying on her deathbed in the closing act of the opera, Violetta is racked with pain and suffering from the terminal phases of her tuberculosis. Dr. Grenvil enters, sits quietly next to her, and takes her pulse. An experienced physician of his time, the doctor no doubt feels the irregular, deathly weak pulse of a patient dying of TB because minutes later he whispers to Violetta's attendant: "Her consumption leaves her only a few hours to live" (Verdi 1962, 326). However, from Dr. Grenvil's actions, it is clear that he understands, and identifies with, his young patient's suffering and fear. Knowing that he cannot treat Violetta medically, the doctor offers her hope, kindness, and affection.

DOCTOR:

Coraggio adunque . . .   Don't be afraid, then . . .
la convalescenza   convalescence isn't
non è lontana . . .   far off . . .

VIOLETTA:

Oh! la bugia pietosa ai   Ah! doctors may tell a
medici è concessa! . . .   compassionate lie! . . .

DOCTOR (*squeezing
her hand*):

Addio . . . a più tardi!   Good-bye . . . till later!
                             (Verdi 1962, 325–26)

Dr. Grenvil has lied to Violetta about her imminent death, and intuitively she is aware of this. Still, this scene is touching and poignant, conveying the sense that the doctor and his patient feel respect, affection, and empathy for each other. Indeed, Dr. Grenvil's empathy for Violetta is so strong that during her climactic death scene at the end of this act, the doctor literally becomes one of the mourning family members.

In this act, Dr. Grenvil is the quintessential empathic physician who, because of his ability to identify with his patient's pain and suffering, has helped her during her death. However, *only* in the context of pre-antibiotic medicine, when there were no adequate medical therapies and little scientific knowledge about tuberculosis, are Dr. Grenvil's actions both appropriate and admirable. In fact, Dr. Grenvil's relative inaction and his misleading statements to Violetta about her illness, which seem so profoundly kind and correct in the context of the mid-nineteenth century, would be malpractice in the 1990s.

For the physician, empathic action is restricted—and enhanced—by scientific knowledge. If Violetta's death scene took place in the 1990s, Dr. Grenvil would have to act very differently to be a responsible and caring physician. Although it would still be acceptable for him to identify with a young, beautiful woman who has a serious infectious disease, he could not let his empathy for his patient's suffering interfere with the appropriate scientific treatment of her illness. In today's world, Dr. Grenvil would be *required* to hospitalize Violetta immediately, place her on any and all appropriate life-saving technology, and treat her with aggressive antibiotic therapy because theoretically her tuberculosis could be reversible.

As scientific knowledge about various diseases progresses over time, it is inevitable that conflicts will arise between previously held convictions about appropriate empathic care in the doctor-patient relationship and the newer scientific information. The more rapidly new scientific knowledge accumulates, the more likely it is that significant conflicts will develop between old and new methods of medical care. The challenge for the modern physician is to *continuously integrate* the newest scientific discoveries into a previously established empathic doctor-patient relationship.

One of the most important examples of an ongoing conflict between previous doctor-patient relationships and new scientific discoveries has occurred in child psychiatry during the last decade. A revolution in the neurobiological sciences has led to a new neurobiological interpretation of many of the serious "mental" illnesses in children and adolescents. This revolution has occurred so rapidly that there is now a severe transitional conflict between older forms of therapy based on psychodynamic and psychoanalytic theories and the newer models based on verifiable, reproducible, scientific evidence. Many health care workers using the older methods have genuine empathy for individuals who suffer from serious psychiatrically defined illnesses and, like Dr. Grenvil, strongly believe that they are acting in the patients' best interests. Empathic doctor-patient relationships must always be evaluated in the light of current scientific knowledge, however. Let us examine the nature of this conflict.

There is now sufficient data to document that many serious childhood "psychiatric" illnesses—including, for example, autism and other pervasive developmental disorders, bipolar disorder, major depressive disorder, obsessive-compulsive disorder, Tourette's syndrome, schizophrenia, anxiety disorders, and attention deficit hyperactivity disorder—are physical illnesses characterized by significant neuroanatomical and neurochemical abnormalities (Peschel et al. 1992). These neurobiological disorders (NBD) are now defined and understood according to the reproducible scientific observations relevant to each disorder. This new data base represents a significant and rapid departure from traditional views of childhood "mental" illnesses. More important, the new treatment approaches for each of these severe physical illnesses called NBD must be based on scientific models and principles, instead of on opinion, theory, belief, and a few anecdotal experiences.

Inevitably, within the institutions of our society that must care for children and adolescents with severe NBD—including the medical profession, educational and legal systems, and governmental agencies—there has been much resistance to the new NBD models. In a false framework of "caring for" and even being "empathic" to these ill children and youth, these institutions continue to ignore, and to fail to integrate into their policies and treatment programs, the irrefutable neuroanatomic and neurochemical data about NBD.

Many of the nonpharmacologic forms of clinical therapy in child psychiatry—for example, psychoanalysis, psychotherapy, psychodynamic therapy, milieu therapy, and family therapy—have not been investigated scientifically. Instead, they rely almost exclusively on anecdotal data, theory, or opinion. There are neither prospective trials nor a significant body of retrospective data to support the use of these therapies for patients with NBD. On the other hand, neuropharmacological therapy for NBD has been evaluated with modern clinical studies that involve either prospective randomized trials or large retrospective data bases.

The Results of Therapy Based on Nonscientific Models

A number of studies have attempted to assess the true clinical efficacy of psychoanalytical and psychodynamic therapies in both children and adults:

1. A study of 600 boys (average age = 10 years) who were judged likely to become delinquent were randomly assigned to either a "no treatment" control group or a "treatment" group that participated in regular psychoanalytic sessions for more than five years. At regular follow-ups—at three years, between five and eleven years, and at thirty years—there was no demonstrable benefit in the treatment group. In fact, the treated group had a worse overall outcome in terms of repeated criminal activity than the untreated control group (Torrey 1992).

2. A clinical trial of intensive individualized psychotherapy for patients with schizophrenia in two Boston hospitals found no therapeutic benefit from such treatment (Klerman 1990).

3. A follow-up study of severely depressed, hospitalized patients treated with

intensive psychotherapy found no evidence for the efficacy for such therapy (Klerman 1990).

4. Of nine reports on nearly 400 children with attention deficit hyperactivity disorder (ADHD), not one demonstrated any benefit from psychotherapy (Klein 1987, 1215–24).

In sharp contrast to the lack of proven efficacy for nonscientific therapies, substantial clinical data for pharmacologic therapy offer overwhelming evidence that such therapy is efficacious.

The Results of Pharmacotherapy Based on Scientific Models

By contrast, a number of studies have confirmed the efficacy of scientific therapies:

1. From a total of twenty-two clinical reports on the use of neuroleptics in patients with schizophrenia, sixteen (73 percent) demonstrated a clear benefit from the use of neuroleptics either in the course of the disease or in the patient's quality of life. Collectively these studies, which included thousands of individuals, demonstrated that patients recover sooner and remain stable longer with the use of neuroleptics (Wyatt 1991, 133–63).

2. For patients with obsessive-compulsive disorder (OCD), fourteen separate prospective randomized clinical trials have all demonstrated the efficacy of clomipramine (Anafranil) (Peschel et al. 1992, 25–28).

3. For children with conduct disorder, there are now two randomized clinical trials demonstrating the efficacy of lithium therapy (Peschel et al. 1992, 59–63).

4. From a total of ninety-five prospective clinical trials, sixty-nine (73 percent) showed a statistically significant benefit compared to a placebo for the use of one of the heterocyclic antidepressants in patients with major depressive disorder (Brotman et al. 1987, 1031–40).

5. A review of five randomized prospective trials and one retrospective study on more than 200 children with ADHD showed that all six studies demonstrated that treatment with methylphenidate (Ritalin) improved the children's social behavior and interactions with adults (Klein 1987, 1215–24).

This review offers overwhelming evidence that scientific approaches based on modern neurobiological principles are efficacious in improving the lives of children and adults with NBD. The lack of demonstrable benefit for psychoanalytic and psychodynamic forms of therapy in serious NBD is striking. Even so, within child psychiatry there is still an ongoing conflict centered on the use of psychodynamic and psychoanalytical theories versus a more modern neuroscientific approach. This conflict highlights the importance of defining empathic treatment approaches within the context of current scientific knowledge. One cannot *appropriately* identify with the suffering of patients if one remains isolated from, or chooses to ignore, the latest scientific discoveries.

The Lack of Empathy Based on Ignorance

Prejudice—derived for the Latin *prae-*, "before," and *judicium*, "judgment"—implies prejudgment. It is important to understand the prejudicial role that empathy may play in health care due to ignorance about certain illnesses.

It has become socially acceptable to openly discuss only two kinds of serious NBD: major depression and bipolar disorder. As a result, several well-known writers, entertainers, and other professionals have written books or appeared on television talk shows to share personal information about their struggles with these NBD. No doubt, this kind of open discussion contributes to a better understanding of these two illnesses. Yet how often do any of these forums that reach millions of people advance an understanding of other serious NBD, despite the fact that all NBD have a similar underlying pathophysiology rooted in neurochemical or neuroanatomical abnormalities? Open discussions about the biological underpinnings of, and human beings' suffering from, the many other NBDS are extremely rare. Inevitably, such a prejudicial approach results in a *selective empathy* for patients with certain NBDS (bipolar and major depressive disorder), but a glaring lack of empathy for patients with other serious NBDS, including schizophrenia, OCD, and so on.

No profession exemplifies the phenomenon of selective empathy more clearly than the medical profession itself. I (R.E.P.) have personally observed many physicians make the most brutally cruel, insensitive remarks about patients with certain kinds of NBDS such as schizophrenia, anxiety disorders, and obsessive-compulsive disorder. Yet these same physicians often exhibit a caring, empathic relationship with patients who have other physical illnesses, like pancreatic cancer or metastatic cancer, who are experiencing the loss of independence and life goals. These physicians also appear to understand and empathize with patients suffering from depression. These are all examples of selective empathy, for these *same* physicians will remain distant and detached from many patients with NBD who also have pancreatic cancer or metastatic disease. Indeed, these physicians may even joke about the idiosyncratic "behaviors" of such patients despite the fact that the patients' "behaviors" are behavioral *symptoms* due to their aberrant neuroanatomy or neurochemistry.

On the one hand, most physicians understand the sense of loss, pain, and anxiety experienced by cancer patients. Yet most physicians appear ignorant of the similar sense of loss, pain, and suffering endured by most patients with NBD. Both cancer patients and patients with NBD are suffering from physical illnesses, yet one group is treated with selective empathy. Why?

The single most important answer to the problem of selective empathy for patients with NBD is the lack of knowledge about the physical nature of NBD on the part of most of the general medical profession. An example of some of the latest data on schizophrenia is illuminating.

1. More than 100 separate neuroimaging studies throughout the world have documented neuroanatomical differences between patients with schizophrenia and normal control groups (Peschel et al. 1992, 77–82).

2. In several neuroimaging studies of identical twins when one twin had schizophrenia and the other twin did not, there are consistent neuroanatomical abnormalities in the twin with schizophrenia that are *not* seen in the well twin (Peschel et al. 1992, 77–82; Suddath et al. 1990).

3. The latest neuroimaging studies have confirmed that the neuroanatomical abnormalities seen in schizophrenia are present at the onset of the illness (Peschel et al. 1992, 77–82).

4. A recent randomized clinical trial demonstrates the importance of dysfunction of the serotonin system in some patients with schizophrenia (Silver 1992).

5. A recent study at Harvard University demonstrated that the degree of hypoplasia seen on magnetic resonance imaging (MRI) scans in the left temporal lobe of patients with schizophrenia is directly related to the severity of the symptoms of thought disorder that these patients exhibit. In addition, no such anatomical abnormalities are seen in normal control groups (Shenton et al. 1992).

This *irrefutable* evidence for the underlying neurochemical and neuroanatomical basis for NBD has unfortunately not yet been properly integrated into our medical school curricula. This produces the phenomenon of selective empathy. Although it is true that the ignorance about NBD in the medical profession is only a manifestation of a much larger general problem in our society, such inappropriate selective ignorance and empathy should not exist in a profession dedicated to caring for *all of the physically ill.*

Such selective empathy, of course, is nothing new to the medical profession. Medical practitioners, as well as the public, have exhibited prejudice against persons with various kinds of physical illnesses before scientific knowledge about those diseases was integrated into medical practice and society. To illustrate this point, we will briefly discuss misunderstandings about two diseases—leprosy (Hansen's disease) and cancer. Many other diseases have also been the butt of prejudice, cruelty, misconceptions, and scorn—such as bubonic plague, epilepsy, mental retardation, and auto-immune deficiency syndrome (AIDS).

From biblical times and throughout the Middle Ages, physicians and the public viewed leprosy as a disease caused by moral corruption, often linked to illicit sexual intercourse. Thus, Aretaeus wrote that lepers have an "irresistible and shameless impulse for intercourse" (Brady 1974). Because of such beliefs, patients with leprosy were ostracized—literally cast out—from society. The prejudice against leprosy was so pervasive that for centuries even individuals with "psoriasis, eczema, leukoderma" and other noncontagious skin diseases were exiled from society (Lyons and Petrucelli 1978, 345; Ober 1987, 99–152).

Prior to a more scientific understanding of cancer, patients with malignant diseases were also subjected to unmerciful prejudice. Like leprosy, cancer was often associated in people's minds with illicit sexual intercourse. In the late nineteenth century, "many people thought that cancer was related to venereal disease and that victims should be barred from hospitals (Patterson 1987, 23). In 1884, when Mr. and Mrs. John Jacob Astor offered to completely finance a cancer pavilion for the Woman's Hospital of New York, their offer was rejected, partially because hospital board members "were frightened of having cancer patients in the same facility with other women" (Patterson 1987, 23).

At the present time, it is clear that many patients suffering from the serious physical disorders called NBD—like patients with leprosy and cancer before these diseases were understood and accepted in the light of science—will continue to be accorded the neglected end of selective empathy from the medical profession and our society. In fact, in the 1990s, neurobiological disorders—similar to leprosy and cancer in past eras—are associated, in the public mind at least, with sinfulness and illicit sexual behavior. A 1990 article in *Hospital and Community Psychiatry* reported that a recent survey "found that 71 percent of respondents thought severe mental illness [i.e., NBD] was due to emotional weakness, . . . [and] 35 percent cited sinful behavior" (Judd 1990). Only when the findings of the neuroscience revolution are *completely integrated* into our medical educational systems will such bias and prejudice against human beings with NBD decrease.

Conclusions

Empathy in the doctor-patient relationship is a complex concept, difficult to define, yet easy to recognize, as in the case of Dr. Grenvil in *La Traviata* of 1853. However, for the physician practicing today, the empathic practice of medicine cannot exclude scientific knowledge and treatment: they will enhance the modern physician's expression of empathy.

In the 1990s, empathy accompanied by ignorance or by rejection of the latest scientific findings *is not empathy at all but intellectual and emotional denial.* The result is selective empathy, which respects patients with certain physical illnesses but which scorns, ignores, or blames patients with other physical illnesses. The only defenses against such selective empathy are continuing education and the integration of scientific advances.

For all physicians and other people who resist the rapid changes that new scientific knowledge imposes—and affords—about patients with physical diseases, including NBD, we recommend a scene from the poignant opera *I Pagliacci* by Ruggiero Leoncavallo. In it, Tonio, a physically deformed man who earns his living as a clown-actor, speaks for the millions of physically handicapped human beings who have suffered throughout the ages from the scorn and ignorance of their fellow mortals:

> E voi, piuttosto che le nostre
> povere gabbane d'istrioni,
> le nostr'anime considerate,
> poichè siam uomini di carne e d'ossa,
> e che di quest'orfano mondo
> al pari di voi spiriamo l'aere!

> So ben che difforme, contorto son io;
> che desto soltanto lo scherno e l'orror.
> Eppure ha' l pensero un sogno, un desiò,
> e un palpito il cor!
> Allor che sdegnosa mi passi d'accanto,
> non sai tu che pianto mi spreme il dolor!

> And you, instead of thinking about
> our tawdry clownish clothes,
> think about our souls,
> for we are human beings made of flesh and bones,
> and, just like you, we breathe
> the air of this orphan world!

> I'm well aware that I'm contorted and deformed,
> that I arouse only horror and scorn.

Yet I have dreams and desires,
and my heart beats!
When you pass by me disdainfully
you do not know that pain is wringing tears from me!
(Leoncavallo 1963)

When dealing with all patients—including those suffering from illnesses that have been or that remain the butt of prejudice—members of the medical profession have a responsibility to remember Tonio's words. What else can the meaning of empathy be?

References

Brady, S. N. 1974. *The Disease of the Soul: Leprosy in Medieval Literature*. Ithaca and London: Cornell University Press.

Brotman, A. W., W. E. Falk, A. J. Gelenberg. 1987. Pharmacologic treatment of acute depressive subtypes. In *Psychopharmacology: The Third Generation of Progress*, ed. H. Y. Meltzer. New York: Raven Press.

Judd, L. L. 1990. Putting mental health on the nation's health agenda. *Hospital and Community Psychiatry*. 41:131–34.

Klein, R. G. 1987. Pharmacotherapy of childhood hyperactivity: An update. In *Psychopharmacology: The Third Generation of Progress*, ed. H. Y. Meltzer. New York: Raven Press.

Klerman, G. L. 1990. The psychiatric patient's right to effective treatment: Implication of Osheroff v. Chestnut Lodge. *American Journal of Psychiatry*. 147:409–18.

Leoncavallo, R. 1963. *I Pagliacci*. Libretto by R. Leoncavallo. Piano-vocal score #45607. New York and London: G. Schirmer.

Lyons, A. S., and R. J. Petrucelli. 1978. *Medicine: An Illustrated History*. New York: Harry N. Abrahams.

Ober, W. B. 1987. Can the leper change his spots?: The iconography of leprosy. In *Bottoms Up! A Pathologist's Essays on Medicine and the Humanities*, by W. B. Ober. Carbondale and Edwardsville: Southern Illinois University Press.

Patterson, J. T. 1987. *The Dread Disease: Cancer and Modern American Culture*. Cambridge, Mass.: Harvard University Press.

Peschel, R. E., and E. R. Peschel. 1985. The tubercular patient in art and in life. *Medical Heritage*. 1:422–33.

Peschel, E. R., R. E. Peschel, C. W. Howe, and J. W. Howe, eds. 1992. *Neurobiological Disorders in Children and Adolescents*. New Directions for Mental Health Services, no. 54. San Francisco: Jossey-Bass.

Shenton, M. E., R. Kikinis, et al. 1992. Abnormalities of the left temporal lobe and thought disorder in schizophrenia: A quantitative magnetic resonance imaging study. *New England Journal of Medicine*. 327:605–12.

Silver, H. 1992. Fluvoxamine improves negative symptoms in treated chronic schizophrenia: An add-on double-blind placebo controlled study. *Biological Psychiatry.*
31:698–704.

Suddath, R. L., G. W. Christison, E. F. Torrey, M. F. Casanova, and D. R. Weinberger.
1990. Anatomical discordant for schizophrenia. *New England Journal of Medicine.*
322:789–94.

Torrey, E. F. 1992. *Freudian Fraud: The Malignant Effect of Freud's Theory on American
Thought and Culture.* New York: Harper Collins.

Verdi, G. 1962. *La Traviata.* Libretto by Piave. Piano-vocal score #133060. New York:
Ricordi. English translations are by Enid Peschel.

Wyatt, R. J. 1991. Neuroleptics and the natural course of schizophrenia. In *New Develop-
ments in the Pharmacologic Treatment of Schizophrenia,* ed. J. M. Kane. Washington,
D.C.: National Institutes of Mental Health, U.S. Department of Health and Human
Services.

Chapter 12
Science, Pedagogy, and the Transformation of Empathy in Medicine

STANLEY JOEL REISER

This chapter explores how empathic understanding in medicine has been adversely affected by the tendency to classify patients into categories of disease. It also examines the related rise of a technologic approach to diagnosis and its effect on the physician's ability to be empathic. Finally, it probes the relationship between students and teachers for clues to the use of empathy in medicine and develops a code of ethics for teaching as a means of reshaping and clarifying this relationship.

The Transmutation of Illness into Disease

When his student Richard Blackmore asked the English physician Thomas Sydenham "to advise me what books I should read to qualify me for practice" Sydenham, without elaborating on its meaning replied, "Read *Don Quixote*, it is a very good book. I read it still" (Dewhurst 1966, 49). The time of this exchange was the seventeenth century, a period when medicine was crossing the border between its philosophic past and its scientific future, with

121

Sydenham himself a crucial agent in the transition. His suggestion to Blackmore points to the high regard physicians of that century placed on understanding their lives. What could a young person know of life? Little, by the measure of experience. Literature, one can surmise, seemed to Sydenham a good remedy for this lack, particularly literature successful in portraying the ambiguities and complexities of life. And where could one better learn of the ambiguities and complexities of life than by immersing oneself in the adventures of the Don? It is thus ironic that Sydenham's greatest clinical achievement, his concept of illness as disease, would begin the process of removing from medicine a concern for personal experience that is embedded in his advice to his student and that forms the essence of empathy.

The degree to which physicians of this period appreciated that illness was the patient's own story can be seen in the existing medical tradition of diagnosing and prescribing through the mails. Here, for example, is a letter a patient wrote to that well-known Dutch physician Hermann Boerhaave:

> Sir,
>
> I am twenty-seven years old, and for about four years last past, any violent action brings on me a difficulty of breathing, which is attended with a cough and spitting, which seldom holds me above half an hour or not so long, if I can spit freely; if I drink any strong spirituous liquor late in the evening, I am awakened frequently in the night with a shortness of breathing, but mostly after malt liquors, and likewise tobacco, any slight cold always aggravates it, and likewise cold weather; when action brings it on me, it is often attended with pain in my head, it has been easier this winter, than it was foregoing ones, and I have been less subject to take cold, which advantage I fancy to have received by taking twelve or fifteen drops of oil of sulfur per Campan in a glass of cold water at night. In my youth I had convulsion fits, and am more subject to this shortness of breath in the winter, than in the summer, I have my health otherwise very well, and a good appetite. (Boerhaave 1745)

Boerhaave sent back a letter that discussed the patient's condition and prescribed appropriate therapy.

Sydenham also followed this tradition of writing cases from the patient's perspective. Yet he was intrigued by a search undertaken in his time by scientific explorers of the biologic world, such as his colleagues in the Royal Society of London. They probed nature to identify and classify plants, establishing their connections to each other through shared characteristics. This search created ever-lengthening lists of species, genera, families, and orders. Sydenham, an astute observer of clinical symptoms, was struck by the notion that, like plants, diseases were discrete entities and could be classified by predisposing traits and characteristic symptoms patients experienced and displayed over time. As he wrote: "To draw a disease in gross is an easy matter. To describe it in its history . . . is far more difficult" (Sydenham 1850, 1). He complained that the categories under which physicians discussed disorders were so broad as to inadequately distinguish among them. Many disorders were confused and placed together under some large common heading. Or distinctions were made between disorders on the basis of a philosophic theory about the nature of illness rather than from an authentic description of their natural characteristics.

Indeed, at this time illnesses were essentially perceived as they were in ancient Greece, as variants of a single disorder, a humoral disruption. One got sick when the body's essential components, the four humors, whose balance constituted health, became unbalanced through the action of environmental, physical, or emotional causes. The physician's task was to diagnose which of the humors had caused the imbalance and to restore the equilibrium state through appropriate therapy. This therapy was not directed at the illness as an entity but rather at the problem of reestablishing humoral balance. In a basic way, each illness was as unique as the patient in which it occurred. The physician treated the illness of the person.

Sydenham continued to believe in the existence of the humors and to accept that the various imbalances among them were the essential cause of illness. He declared, however, that this pathological process was not, as generally conceived, "a confused and disordered effort of Nature thrown down from her proper state" (Sydenham 1850, 1), but that each imbalance constituted a particular event with characteristic symptoms which, when taken together, defined a specific entity. The entity could be named and identified in the people stricken by it. By this reasoning the illnesses of different people could be combined and transformed into specific disease histories. As Sydenham said, "Nature, in the production of disease is uniform and consistent; so much so, that for the same disease in different persons the symptoms are for the most part the same; and the selfsame phenomena you would observe in the sickness of a Socrates you would observe in the sickness of a simpleton" (Sydenham 1850, 1). Such clear definition of diseases would allow physicians to identify specific remedies for them and thereby improve therapy—an important goal Sydenham had for medicine.

Sydenham described these afflictions in portraits that delineated the sequence of symptoms characterizing particular diseases. Here is one such portrait:

RHEUMATISM.

This disease may come on at any time. It is commonest, however, during the autumn, chiefly attacking the young and vigorous. It generally originates in some such cause as the following. The patient has been heated by either some overviolent exercise, or by some other means, and has taken cold upon it. The sad list of symptoms begins with chills and shivers; these are followed immediately by heat, disquietude, thirst, and the other concomitants of fever. One or two days after this (sometimes sooner) the patient is attacked by severe pains in the joints, sometimes in one and sometimes in another, sometimes in his wrist, sometimes in his shoulder, sometimes in the knee—in this last joint oftenest. This pain changes its place from time to time, takes the joints in turns, and affects the one that it attacks last with redness and swelling. Sometimes during the first days the fever and the above-named symptoms go hand in hand; the fever, however, gradually goes off whilst the pain only remains; sometimes, however, it grows worse. . . . There is plenty of the disease now-a-days; and, although it very rarely, when once the fever has been driven off, kills the patient, it is still from the vehemence of the pain, and from its protracted duration, no contemptible distemper. Treat it badly, and it will last for months and years; nay, it will torment a patient throughout his miserable lifetime.

Its violence, indeed, may vary; so that, after the fashion of gout, it may come on at odd times, and in periodic fits. This, too, may happen after the aforesaid pains have been long, violent, and afflicting. Then they may cease of their own accord: the patient, however, shall be a cripple to the day of his death. (Sydenham 1850, 1)

In constructing such disease histories Sydenham identified two types of symptoms: "constant" and "adventitious" ones. The constant phenomena were pathognomonic symptoms that defined the disease entities and were shared by the population afflicted with the disease. The adventitious phenomena were idiosyncratic symptoms unique to each sufferer; these symptoms expressed the differing personalities and responses of individuals to illness. It has been Sydenham's legacy to medicine to elevate the pathognomonic above the idiosyncratic symptoms. The goal of evaluating illness has become the classification of people into delimited categories of diseases. Thus the symptoms that combine patients into populations have become more significant to physicians than the symptoms that separate patients as individuals. This hallmark of modern medicine was a major step in physicians' growing detachment from the unique traits of their patients. It diminished physicians' ability to understand and to identify with the patient's persona and thus reduced their empathic concern.

Technology and Empathy

Physicians appreciate illness through diagnostic techniques they interpose between themselves and patients. These techniques filter evidence, blocking out some of its features, emphasizing others. This selection allows characteristic portraits of illness to be generated. In the early nineteenth century, the characteristic portrait was derived from the comments of patients. It was a narrative of subjective feelings and events. What distinguished the seventeenth- from the nineteenth-century narrative was the significance given to those special features upon which Sydenham had focused. In the nineteenth century, physicians sought to establish a pattern that was diagnostic of a particular disease by focusing on symptoms that were pathognomonic rather than idiosyncratic.

Despite this molding of the patient's story to produce a standardized view of illness (a sign of medicine's progress as a scientific discipline), physicians bemoaned their dependence on the testimony of patients for essential medical facts. Patients seemed untrustworthy. They might forget, distort, or confuse essential evidence and physicians could not know that they were making these errors. Even if physicians were suspicious of the story, they could not usually confirm their misgivings.

This situation was transformed in the nineteenth century by a new set of technologies spearheaded by the stethoscope, introduced in 1819, which was soon followed by the ophthalmoscope, laryngoscope, and gastroscope. These technologies had a common trait—they extended the senses of the physician into the interior of the body. This produced a common result—their findings created physician-drawn portraits of illness that replaced ones derived from the patient's story (Reiser 1978).

Take as an example the ophthalmoscope. What we see with our eyes is highly personal, and we appreciate it in ways others cannot know. Before this new technology appeared, the evaluation of a patient's vision was principally based on subjective accounts of the sensations, shapes, and colors appreciated by the eyes and mind of the patient. The power the ophthalmoscope gave the physician was the power of independent judgment. The instrument permitted an observer to look directly into the eye and view the basic anatomical structures that might be damaged by pathology. This permitted the physician to evaluate the essential parts of the eye without the intervening opinions of the patient. What patients thought, described, or felt about their vision was not considered as significant as what a medical observer saw or did not see in their eyes. This diminished medical reliance, as one doctor put, "on the faltering judgment of the untrained patient, substituting therefore the skill of the expert (Wurdemann 1894, 341).

The instruments of physical diagnosis redirected the physician's attention from a focus on the patient's experiences to a focus on the body's structures. Once again the physician's ability to be empathic in medical relationships was made more difficult, this time by a shift in what was valued as evidence of illness.

The diagnostic technology of twentieth-century medicine has intensified this retreat from an interest in the patient's persona. Its focus remains the physical features of the body and its diseases, and the evidence it generates stated as numbers, graphs, and anatomic images. The portraits of illness that physicians draw with this data remain as impersonal as the ones they constructed from data produced by the instruments of physical diagnosis. But the views created by the new technologies—the images of the X-ray, the graphs of the electrocardiograph, and the numbers of the automated chemical analyzer—place the physician a step further from the patient than those generated by the older technologies. Medical examination with a stethoscope at least required a patient on one end and a doctor on the other. An X-ray of a patient can be taken in the doctor's absence. Thus modern technology introduces an impersonal dimension into the story of illness; it also fosters an ever-growing distance between physicians and patients. They see less of each other, and more of technicians and reports. This is reflected in the average length of a patient's visit with a contemporary physician, which in the United States is twelve minutes (Stoeckle 1987).

The Student-Teacher Relationship in Medicine

The relationship between students and teachers has had an important bearing on the development of empathy in medicine. To understand its beginnings we must turn to the Hippocratic Oath. The Oath is commonly viewed as an ethical code, containing moral principles to guide physicians in their relationships with patients. This is true, but only of its second half. Early in the Oath is a passage focused on the relationship between the student and the teacher of medicine. This part is as significant as the succeeding code. It describes the basis for learning medicine, the norms of conduct practitioners should adopt toward each other, and the terms of association in the entity that we have come to know as a profession. The Oath begins with the famous line: "I swear by Apollo Physician, by Asclepius, by Health, by Panacea and by all the gods and goddesses, making them my witnesses, that I will carry out, according to my ability and judgment, this oath and this indenture." Then comes the passage on the pedagogic relationship in medicine: "To hold my teacher in this art equal to my own parents; to make him partner in my livelihood; when he is in need of money to share mine with him; to consider his family as my own brothers, and to teach them this art, if they want to learn it, without fee or indenture; to impart precept, oral instruction, and all other instruction to my own sons, the sons of my teacher, and to indentured pupils who have taken the physician's oath, but to nobody else" (Jones 1962).

The central theme of the relationship between student and teacher in the Hippocratic Oath is of family. The students relate to teachers as parents, and to colleagues as brothers. Students are given access to knowledge only after promising, by swearing to the Oath, to use it according to the ethical principles it announces. Moreover, they cannot teach what they subsequently learn to anyone who has not also sworn to abide by the ethical canons of the Oath. Teachers are to be cared for by students and helped by them if needed, even to the extent of sharing income. In sum, the Oath establishes strong bonds to ethical precepts and to the relationships between students themselves and student and teacher. These allegiances are meant to prevent physicians from using their status or technology in any way that is self-serving or harmful to patients.

In contemporary times, the student-teacher relationship has not had the standing given to it by the ancient Greeks. Its importance is asserted but its ethical dimension is not focused on and specified. Physicians believe the principal goal of this relationship is the transmission of knowledge. How this is done seems less significant than that it be done. We tolerate a wide variety of teaching behaviors by faculty and by hospital residents if they ultimately result in knowledge acquisition by students.

This policy is short-sighted. How students are treated is as important as the technical facts imparted to them. Both actions are lessons. Treating them as inferiors, as muddled beginners, or as tireless acolytes who must accommodate instructor requests teaches them a lesson that is as significant to subsequent patient care as learning correct drug doses is. The Hippocratic physicians recognized this. They would not impart technical knowledge disconnected from a relational context. Can we ignore the attitudes unwittingly instilled in medical students by instructors who have not recognized that there is a connection between the way they treat students and the way students will treat patients?

Institutions as Educators

Increasingly the lives of medical students and physicians are centered in organizations. They are educated in them, spend much of their working days and nights in them, and express their identity through them. Thus organizations are a significant element of medical life. The missions they establish, the values they hold, and the policies they develop influence the people they instruct and employ.

Unfortunately these institutional activities are neglected as sources of education. The site of instruction is thought to be confined to the classroom or clinic. There the knowledge and role models are encountered that will establish patterns of thought and ethics. Other features of institutional life are believed tangential to influencing what physicians become.

This view is limited. It implies that people construct pedagogic walls in their mind, absorbing classroom lessons that bear on values and actions, and ignoring lessons that come from other parts of the institution. An unkind registrar, an indifferent security guard, an unthoughtful schedule of tuition payments, a relative inattention to student needs from a greater concern for research goals, a policy toward the poor of the community that disregards their needs, treatment of a popular teacher that does not reflect significant contributions given to student learning and life, inadequate policies toward minorities or gender issues—the list of possible institutional behaviors can be long. But do they count as education? They do. Why should students believe the rhetoric of the classroom more than the actions of the institution housing it? Which says more about what really counts?

Institutional policy on the relative value given to teaching, research, and clinical service is also significant in setting a moral tone. It is widely acknowledged that research counts more heavily in the decision to promote a professor than success in teaching or clinical service. The allocation of faculty time among these pursuits is inevitably influenced by such an institutional preference.

Taken together, institutional policies give students profound lessons about what matters. Institutions must ask themselves: Do their policies teach the goal of valuing people? Do their actions encourage an empathic perspective in their students?

Creating Empathic Attitudes in Medicine

During the 1970s, I joined John D. Stoeckle, professor of medicine and director of the primary care division at Massachusetts General Hospital, to teach medical students the technique and art of the clinical interview. Using an unobtrusive video camera and recorder, medical students were taped eliciting from patients the story of their illness. These recordings were played back to students and instructors, who reviewed and studied the exchanges that occurred.

The results were interesting. First-year medical students often elicited the true purposes for which the appointment was sought and gained a comprehensive picture of the factors influencing patient symptoms, behaviors, needs, and requests. They did this without having much idea about the clinical significance of the complaints they heard.

Clinical understanding was the preserve of the third-year students whom we recorded. Their histories were filled with the knowledge of pathology. But often they were not as good as first-year students in gaining an accurate and comprehensive view of what bothered the patient, or what living with the illness was like. The third-year students were not after the special events that shape a person's illness: theirs was a quest for disease. The video captured them, antennae out for pathognomonic symptoms, cutting off discourse that diverted attention from tracking the symptom cluster that classified the ailment into an established diagnostic category.

The disparate behavior of first- and third-year medical students was the result of education. First-year students listened to the story of illness. Third-year medical students strove to write a story of disease. For them the disease was the thing: classification, or merging the current patient with preceding patients, was their objective.

Understanding each patient's individuality should be the goal of physicians. Classification into diagnostic groups must be seen as a first, not a final step in the process of knowing. Classification gives physicians invaluable data about those who suffered from similar problems in the past and the outcome of various therapies on them. With knowledge in hand of the similarities between a given patient and others, the physician should take medical inquiry to the next step—establishing how the patient is different from this linked population. From these facts, therapy appropriate to human uniqueness can be developed, and a true empathic connection can be established between physician and patient.

Technologic evidence will form a portion of the facts of patient care. Here physicians must take a more critical view of its reach and limits. Technologic facts derive their scientific authenticity largely because they are stated in numerical, graphical, and pictorial terms. This gives such evidence a quality of objectivity, meaning that in their production, the facts have been rendered free of human bias. This belief neglects several features of technologic evidence. First, the principal advantage of such evidence is its quality of precision. A statement of the hemoglobin content of blood as 13.5 is more precise than its visual estimate as hues in the nail bed (a rosy pink, for example), the yardstick in place before the appearance of a chemical test with a numeric result. Such precision allows clinicians to transmit data from person to person without loss of content. The value 13.5 has a common meaning to medical observers: the phrase "rosy pink" does not.

We often mistake precision for accuracy, however. Data may be precise but inaccurate. Thus an auto-analyzer performing the hemoglobin test on a sample of blood may produce the same result for each of 100 trials. But if the machine was not calibrated appropriately at the start of the day, that answer will be wrong 100 times. The birthplace and form of evidence do not define its value.

This brings us to the place of the patient's story, the history, in clinical medicine. It is the main source of knowing illness in ways that technology cannot fathom. Only the patient's story gives human meaning to the facts elicited by technology. The test can tell the blood count is low, the patient can tell what it means to live with it. Only patients can tell us such things—technology cannot. To recapture an ability to feel and thus know, at least partly, how a patient experiences a given illness and to receive critical evidence about what to do therapeutically, the physician must listen to the patient, and question, and listen again.

The ability to enter the patient's life, the essence of empathy, is practiced less often than the ability to enter into the patient's body through medical technology. This imbalance must and can be corrected. Physicians need both kinds of knowledge. Technologic knowledge creates a portrait of being. Empathic knowledge creates a portrait of meaning. Linked together the two views re-create as nearly as possible the person who is the patient.

To pursue a comprehensive analysis of an illness, the physician must feel predisposed. This predisposition is greatly influenced by received medical education. A technologic learning, provided at the expense of concern for the person who is the learner, is less likely to produce a physician who will devote the time needed to synthesize the being and meaning aspects of a medical evaluation. The professor or resident physician who describes with some pride how he or she pushed students to their physical and intellectual limits to impart clinical and technical excellence and points with a sense of achievement to the outcome has not really evaluated it. Ends produced at the expense of means that ignore essential values in medicine—such as in this instance the do-no-harm precept—are ends purchased at too high a price.

The gains of science should not be sought at the expense of humaneness—not anywhere in life, but especially not in medicine, this remarkable social institution whose members must daily prove themselves worthy of a crucial trust: that they will never take advantage of the vulnerability that is the hallmark of the patients who appear before them. Recall that the Hippocratic doctors, whose values shaped the practice of medicine as we know it, would not teach medicine to those who would not first agree to abide by an ethical code. They know what we should remember: that without the empathy gained through ethical concern, the agents and knowledge of medicine are dangerous and untrustworthy.

The humanistic dimension of medical teaching is thus as significant as its scientific aspect. The two should be regarded as equal parts of the medical whole. To set forth a group of values that can help define the obligations of teachers and students, I have written an ethical code:

A Code of Ethics for Teaching Medicine
1. Teachers should treat students as they wish them to treat patients.
2. There are two main branches of learning in medicine. One is scientific, the other humanistic. Each must be taught with equal commitment and knowledge.
3. Scientific learning is necessary so that students will not harm the patients they treat and will have an ability to create new knowledge. Humanistic learning is needed for the same reasons.
4. A teacher should be an educator and a friend to the student. As educator the teacher seeks intellectual growth. As friend, the teacher fosters the security to attain this growth.
5. What are the duties of teachers to students? They are many but three predominate: *Candor*—about students and self. Without an honest appraisal of their efforts, students cannot know where improvement is needed. Without an honest revealing of their own limits, teachers present a false image of the limits of knowing. *Trust*—bestowing trust on learners encourages their efforts to become reliable, a quintessential value of the practitioner in the clinic or the laboratory. *Respect*—for the diversity, effort, accomplishment, viewpoints, and limits of students. This gives them a dignity essential for growth and self-esteem.
6. What are the duties of students to teachers? Here too three stand out: *Reciprocity*—recognizing the need to reward efforts to teach with a commitment to learn. *Honesty*—in acquiring knowledge and admitting where more learning is needed. *Openness*—being receptive and giving a fair hearing to ideas.
7. A teacher should strive to create a humane environment toward students in the institution within which they learn. Humane rules and personnel foster an atmosphere within which the values of kindness and forbearance are transmitted.
8. Academic teachers are not the only sources of learning for students. Institutional personnel also give them lessons about respect and concern for others through the policies they follow and the actions they take. In this regard they too are educators.
9. Teaching should be valued by academic faculty. It combines responsibilities for the well-being of the students entrusted to their care and for knowledge

honestly appraised and carefully transmitted. This dual responsibility for people and for learning is central to the mission of medical institutions.

10. These institutions in turn should esteem teaching as the bridge between knowledge and action, and an art and science equal in worth and complexity to research and service to patients.

References

Boerhaave, H. 1745. *Medical Correspondence . . .* London: John Nourse.

Dewhurst, K., ed. 1966. *Dr. Thomas Sydenham (1624–1689)*, quoting from Blackmore, *A Treatise upon the Smallpox*, 1723. Berkeley and Los Angeles: University of California Press.

Jones, W. H. S., trans. 1962. Hippocrates: The oath. In *Hippocrates*, vol. 1. Cambridge: Harvard University Press.

Reiser, S. J. 1978. *Medicine and the Reign of Technology*. New York: Cambridge University Press.

Stoeckle, J. D. 1987. The structure: Ground rules for the doctor-patient relationship. In *Encounters between Doctors and Patients*, ed. J. D. Stoeckle. Cambridge: The MIT Press.

Sydenham, T. 1850. Medical observations concerning the history and the cure of acute diseases. In *The Works of Thomas Sydenham, M.D.*, trans. R. G. Latham, vol. 1. London: New Sydenham Society.

Wurdemann, H. V. 1894. The status of skiascopy. *Journal of the American Medical Association*. 23:341.

Part Three
The Theory of
Empathy

This final section provides some theoretical considerations of empathy. For Joseph S. Alpert and Helle Mathiasen, literature and art are the wellsprings of empathy. An aphorism from Herodotus, "My sufferings have been my lessons," brings them to divide empathy into *empirical* and *natural* forms. The first comes from suffering in this world, the second from a willingness to enter into the world of another. The records of human thought provide a treasure chest for those "health care professionals" who would be empathic. King Lear learns empathy for his servant only after he has lost his royal power. Chekhov's doctor who does not suffer with his patients might well be working on our modern wards; only when he loses his power and becomes a patient does he learn to appreciate empathy. Like LeVasseur and Vance, Alpert and Mathiasen want empathy to be more than a tool or a technique. It must be felt: that vast, formless, irresistible sense of being at one with the world that seizes us from time to time; the music of a celebration may bring us close to it.

Rita Charon suggests how patients' stories may steer us as close to empathy as great literature can. What others might call "illness," the story of the patient, she renames "narrative knowledge"; the science and reason we bring to a "case" she calls "logico-scientific knowledge." In rejecting narrative, which concerns the motivations and consequences of human action, as recent immigrants from the world of mysticism, modern physicians take pride in emphasizing their logico-scientific work. Yet if so many problems that bring people to physicians have social, economic, and spiritual origins, physicians cannot ignore the stories that alone can help them to deliver empathic care to the sick.

Although empathy was largely ignored by Freud and those who followed, the past few decades have seen a growing interest among psychiatrists. Jodi Halpern argues strongly against the idea that empathy is purely intellectual, that the good physician can empathize without actually feeling anything. Physicians of the 1950s may have idealized detachment, but Halpern exalts feeling as part of empathy and agrees that it is far more than just a tool. In separating emotions from neurophysiological reactions, Halpern wants to restore the mind as more than the brain. Long ago, Leibnitz pointed out that even if we could see the workings of the brain laid out in some huge model, we would still not know where to locate charity, love, or hate. Emotions move people in different ways because people emphasize different aspects of reality; transference and counter-transference interfere with the ways physicians manage their emotions, she says. Listening with curiosity she finds essential to the resonance that brings empathy, helping doctors to practice more effective, not just more enjoyable, medicine.

Peter Kramer, a practicing psychiatrist in Providence, locates empathy as much in the patient as in the physician. For him, empathy is always an interaction, by those who learn early in life to be "adept at amplifying small interpersonal cues." For him, too, empathy is more than a tool or a source of information; following Heinz Kohut and Harry Stack Sullivan, he finds that empathy may unlock the patient's healing powers, partly by restoring self-confidence. Some readers may find therapeutic empathy more intuitive than persuasive, more interpretation than intent, but for me his delightful chapter opens up a special aspect of empathy.

H. M. S.

Chapter 13
Lessons in Empathy: Literature, Art, and Medicine

HELLE MATHIASEN
AND JOSEPH S. ALPERT

"Who taught you all this, Doctor?"
The reply came promptly:
"Suffering."
—Albert Camus, *The Plague*

"My sufferings have been my lessons" (*ta de moi pathemata mathemata gegone*), writes the Greek historian Herodotus. Two words in this phrase apply to physicians dealing, as all physicians do, with suffering patients. The first word is *pathemata*, derived from *pathema*, meaning "anything that befalls one: a suffering, calamity, misfortune" (Liddell and Scott 1966, 583). The second Greek term important to physicians is *mathemata*, from *mathema*, a lesson, knowledge, science. This etymology focuses attention on the thesis of this essay, namely that a knowledge or science of suffering can be acquired. Is it true, as Herodotus states, that the science of suffering, or empathy, can only be learned or known by one who has suffered? Can only a person who has suffered be in a state of *empathes*, that is, "in a state of emotion . . . much affected by or at a thing?" (Liddell and Scott 1966, 254). This is probably true, judging from the huge amount of testimony from literature available to us, whether it be the memoirs we can pick up in airports, composed by survivors of illness and their friends, or the fictional representations of suffering found in established writers such as Shakespeare, Chekhov, Williams, Camus, and Moerch. But it is not necessary for health professionals to suffer mental or physical pain in order to acquire empathy. They can learn about this feeling vicariously through literature and art.

Empathy, or the ability to be affected by an event not one's own, is clearly a desirable quality for a physician to have; however, not all physicians show this capacity. They may never have learned it at home, nor in school nor in medical training. If Herodotus is correct, physicians who have suffered will resemble other people in being more empathetic than those who have not themselves suffered. Should we then require physicians who have lived relatively painless lives—defined by vague standards—to expose themselves to suffering? Should such a health care worker choose to submit to horrible suffering? Not at all. Denial is a rational response to suffering. Instead of suffering, then, a physician may learn empathy through the enjoyment of literature and art.

At this point, it is useful to distinguish between two kinds of empathy: empirical empathy and natural empathy. For the sake of clarity, we will use examples from accomplished writers to illustrate these two different states of mind. Herodotus alludes to empirical empathy when he describes the didactic value of his own sufferings. He has suffered, in body and mind; because he has a philosophical bent, he is able to translate his experiences into valuable lessons. A personal crisis, such as a physical or mental illness, can create empirical empathy in an individual who has not been particularly sensitive to the pain of other people. However, a personal crisis does not occur on demand, nor does everyone profit from suffering. On the contrary, severe mental and physical agony can deaden the feelings. It may actually be exceptional individuals who grow into empathy through their own pain. Indeed, sometimes suffering is just pain, with no lesson to follow. But in the case of empirical empathy, a lesson *is* drawn from one's own suffering: one learns to feel for others and to show this feeling.

The second kind of empathy, natural empathy, is found more often than not in most people. It does not require personal suffering, only a willingness to suspend disbelief, to use the imagination, and to enter into the world of the other. Medical education and training can encourage an understanding of both empirical and natural empathy by making available to students, interns, and residents courses and discussion groups that focus on important works of literature and art.

Shakespeare's *King Lear* offers an excellent example of empirical empathy, but not one that anyone would care to repeat. Shakespeare chooses a story about a foolish old man who wants to retire and have his children take care of him and his property; even though he has abdicated, King Lear still wants to be revered as a powerful father and king. The point of the play is that without his property, the king, even the king, is nobody. He is no better than his Fool. Externals do not make him great; they are just trappings of power. King Lear's slow awakening to this reality leads to his lesson in empathy. This begins when his deprivations in the storm cause his mind to blur the conventional distinction between King and Fool. When his own pain opens his mind to perceive the pain of another, King Lear's empathy begins to emerge. But, cruelly, King Lear has to lose his mind to gain wisdom. Rejected by his greedy daughters Goneril and Regan, King Lear and his Fool stand on the heath, blasted by the winds and pounded by the rains of a fearful storm. Lear says to his Fool:

> My wits begin to turn.
> Come on, my boy. How dost, my boy? Art cold?
> I am cold myself. Where is this straw, my fellow?
> The art of our necessities is strange,
> That can make vile things precious. Come, your hovel.
> Poor Fool and knave, I have one part in my heart
> That's sorry yet for thee. (*King Lear*, act 3, scene 2, ll. 68–73)

King Lear feels for the Fool. He is learning that his Fool suffers as he does. But Lear's empathy comes at an outrageous cost. The suffering King has lost his kingdom and family; however, he has gained human knowledge and feelings. He now shows kindness to the Fool; he asks forgiveness from his good daughter Cordelia. Lear's sufferings have enable him to feel for and give to others. But then he dies.

Empirical empathy, the positive outcome of painful experience, cannot be better illustrated than by *King Lear*. But there is such a sense of loss at the end of Shakespeare's tragedy that King Lear's torments seem excessive. Lear's empirical empathy lesson costs him his family, his sanity, and his life.

For another powerful image of empirical empathy relevant to health care professionals, we can turn to the work of physician-writer Anton Chekhov. In his famous story "Ward Six," Chekhov employs his artistry to illustrate an example of a doctor learning empirical empathy. Chekhov accomplishes this using a reversal technique similar to Shakespeare's. King Lear becomes an old fool—King reverts to Fool; Chekhov's doctor reverts to being a patient. In both cases, the empathy lesson almost annihilates the suffering learner. And the fruits of the lesson are puny. In fact, both Shakespeare and Chekhov seem to wish to punish their protagonists for extraordinary vanity and negligence. The authors do not allow their characters to derive more than a passing benefit from their agony.

In "Ward Six," Chekhov presents Dr. Ragin. In charge of a mental ward, Ward Six, Dr. Ragin is unable to empathize with his patients. Overwhelmed by his job, Dr. Ragin neglects his medical tasks in favor of philosophical conversations with the brightest patient in the ward, Gromov. However, when Gromov tells the doctor about his sufferings, Dr. Ragin brushes him off, quoting the Stoic Marcus Aurelius and thus dismissing Gromov's pain as something that he should be able to meditate away. To Dr. Ragin, pain exists only in the mind; at this stage of life, his own life calm and comfortable, Dr. Ragin does not suffer. Gromov accuses him, "You may despise suffering, but you catch your finger in the door and I bet you'll scream your head off" (Chekhov 1974, 50). Ragin is skeptical. Through another doctor's trickery, Dr. Ragin suddenly becomes just another patient in Ward Six. Having lost his status as a physician, Dr. Ragin now has to suffer a beating by the ward caretaker, Nikita, who has been beating the patients regularly. This is Chekhov's precise rendering of Dr. Ragin's empathy lesson:

> It was horrible. Ragin lay down and held his breath—terrified, awaiting another blow. He felt as if someone had stuck a sickle in him and twisted it a few times inside his chest and guts. He bit the pillow in his pain and clenched his teeth. Then suddenly, a fearful thought past all bearing flashed through the chaos of his mind: that just such a pain must be the daily lot, year in and out, of these men who loomed before him like black shadows in the moonlight. How could it be that for twenty years and more he had ignored that—and ignored it willfully? He had not known pain, he had no conception of it, so this wasn't his fault. And yet, his conscience proved as tough and obdurate as Nikita, flooding him from head to heels with an icy chill. (*Ward Six*, 68)

In Dr. Ragin's case, empathy comes too late. His suffering does not redeem him nor anyone else. Shakespeare's old king and Chekhov's physician profit only briefly from their lessons in empathy. The harshness of their experience kills both characters. Their empathy lessons through role reversal are painful to watch.

Though it may be a sure road to empathy to "expose [ourselves] to feel what wretches feel," as King Lear advises other kings to do, such exposure is not included in medical education (*King Lear*, act 3, scene 4, l. 34). The risk of such teaching runs high. Moreover, it is unusual to cultivate pain and disease; after all, the whole purpose of medical training is to alleviate suffering. It is sane to cultivate health. Juvenal's *Mens sana in corpore sano* is the familiar Latin saying that prescribes a healthy mind in a healthy body. King Lear is sick in both body and mind. He barely recovers after his great suffering. Dr. Ragin suffers a stroke.

These literary examples are instructive in defining empirical empathy, but a vicarious *Einfühlung* suffices for most of us.

Our tradition tells us, and we know from the small and large experiences of suffering that we have had, that suffering may indeed enable us to empathize. Such empathy can enable physicians to feel for the patient, to put themselves in the patient's place, to glimpse for a moment what it is like to be confined there, on the other side of competence and daylight.

Through their appeal to the imagination, literature and art enable the reader and viewer to experience the point of view and the sensations of another human being. When the subject of art is illness or suffering, the imaginative experience of it can bring the viewer closer to helping the other suffering entity. Through literature and art, students and healers can acquire enlightenment about a painful or joyous event in the life of another. If they are turned into empathy lessons, some works of literature and art can become part of the healing process benefiting both doctor and patient.

However, empathy requires a basic ingredient in the learner: an interest in humankind. The physician-writer William Carlos Williams points out how the medical profession enhances the opportunity for human study. In his *Auto-biography*, he writes, "Was I not interested in man? There the thing was, right in front of me. I could touch it, smell it. It was myself, naked, just as it was, without a lie telling itself to me in its own terms" (Williams 1967, 357). Williams emphasizes the revelation of common humanity in the doctor-patient encounter. In this best of all possible worlds described by Williams, the patient is not the other, nor a lower being, but rather your fellow. When facing a gravely ill patient, the empathetic physician might silently exclaim, "There, but for the grace of God, go I." And this understanding could make the doctor treat the patient better.

The philosopher Edith Stein describes linguistically what takes place in a situation of empathy. Instead of suffering or pain, she chooses the feelings of joy to illustrate her point about the existential nature of empathy. The emotion of joy is experienced differently by different individuals, she writes:

> And it is also possible for us to be joyful over the same event, though not filled with exactly the same joy. Joyfulness may be more richly accessible to the others, which difference I grasp empathically. I em-pathically arrive at the "sides" of joyfulness constructed in my own joy. This ignites my joy, and only now is there complete coincidence with what is emphasized. If the same thing happens to others, we empa-thically enrich our feeling so that "we" now feel a different joy from "I," "you," and "he" in isolation. But "I," "you," and "he" are retained

in "we." A "we," not an "I," is the subject of the empathizing. Not through the feeling of oneness, but through empathizing, do we experience others. The feeling of oneness and the enrichment of our own experience become possible through empathy. (Stein 1970, 17)

Through empathy, we do not become the other, but as Williams says, we become like the other: "It was myself," in pain or joy. A case could be constructed where the physician would feel joy at a patient's recovery, but certainly a joy different from the patient's own. As Stein says, "A 'we,' not an 'I,' is the subject of the empathizing." More commonly said today, "I share your joy/ sadness. I know I am not you and you are not me, but we share an experience, and thus become we."

With the increased professionalization and specialization of literature and medicine, however, this kind of communication has been lacking on the theoretical and practical level. This state of affairs was pointed out years ago by the scientist and writer C. P. Snow, when he coined the phrase "the two cultures" to designate science and the arts. What Snow said then about the lack of understanding between science and literature still holds:

> The clashing point of two subjects, two disciplines, two cultures—of two galaxies, so far as that goes—ought to produce creative chances. In the history of mental activity that has been where some of the breakthrough came. The chances are there now. But they are there, as it were, in a vacuum, because those in the two cultures can't talk to each other. (Snow 1981, 16)

This insight receives ample support if one takes a look at the professional journals for medicine and literature. The professional languages of the scientist and the humanist are specialized and more or less unintelligible to those outside the profession. Therefore it may not be literature or art professors who should teach health workers empathy through literature and art. Perhaps those who are to teach empathy need training in both science and the humanities. For it is true that in their theoretical approaches to human experience scientists and humanists do not communicate easily. This failure to understand is a microcosmic reflection of a macrocosmic predicament, the universal communication gap between all people. It is this galactic silence that increases human suffering, in this our inhuman condition, where "Life is short, the art long, opportunity fleeting, experience treacherous, judgment difficult." However, bringing together literature, art, and medicine on an existential basis recovers the original purpose of learning in the Western cultural tradition, namely to focus on the individual human life well lived in all its concreteness.

Michel de Montaigne discourses on this topic in his essay "On the Education of Children": "For it seems to me that the first lessons in which we should steep his [the student's] mind must be those that regulate his behavior and his senses, that will teach him to know himself and to die well and live well" (Montaigne 1973, 21). Montaigne's goal is moral education. Empathy is a moral value; it is a good thing to have. Empathy with others may even teach us about ourselves.

The teaching and learning of values such as empathy can occur through art and literature. But neither literary criticism nor medical research now educate in these matters. In the professional realm, the study of empathy seems confined to the fields of philosophy, psychology, social work, and nursing. However, literature and art of high artistic quality can educate in empathy any physician who is receptive, thereby enriching the healing action resulting from knowledge of others and knowledge of self.

Many artists promote the reader's or spectator's full comprehension of the character and situation of their work. If this vicarious experience occurs, then galactic hopelessness can perhaps be replaced with a feeling of shared humanity on this planet; perhaps life can acquire greater meaning when lived collectively. On the aesthetic value of a shared and ordinary humanity, we can again turn to Montaigne: "The most beautiful lives, to my mind, are those that conform to the common human pattern, with order, but without miracle and without eccentricity" (Montaigne 1973, 136). Specialization in the arts and sciences may further the profession but may not furnish help in living the good life.

Contemporary medical thinking considers empathy a valuable tool for the physician. Possibly this has come down to us from the Greeks, as in Hippocrates' precept, "First, do no harm." Empathy reminds the healer to heal with the least amount of pain to the patient. Empathy, including an interest in humanity and a sense of fellowship with others, can enable the physician to imagine what the patient is experiencing, without becoming the patient.

Through their appeal to the imagination, literature and art can be useful in developing empathy; they can even be enjoyable. When the subject of literature and art is illness or suffering, the vicarious experience of such fictional creations can bring you closer to an understanding of the other's situation and thereby closer to helping the other suffering human. Through literature and art, medical students and medical practitioners can vicariously participate in another life, but without undergoing such crushing pain as either King Lear or Dr. Ragin. Empirical empathy is painful, even if we only read about it. Natural empathy demonstrated in art and literature is truly enjoyable.

Two different examples from literature will serve to illustrate natural empathy. The characters showing natural empathy do not have to lose their minds to gain wisdom; their feelings for themselves encompass their ability to feel for others. The first example, from Camus's *The Plague*, shows a fictional care-giver's empathy in a crisis setting, during an epidemic of bubonic plague. The second example, from Moerch's novel *Winter's Child*, shows a physician behaving empathetically in a hospital environment. In both stories, the characters portraying natural empathy function well in their jobs as medical professionals. Their feelings of empathy for their patients also make the characters likable; and their empathy, rather than destroying them, enhances their professional lives. Studying and discussing such stories and carrying these vicarious lessons of natural empathy away from Camus and Moerch is not an arduous task. In addition, these stories not only help to define empathy, they also teach us how empathetic people behave.

In Camus's classic novel *The Plague*, the narrator, Dr. Rieux, is naturally empathetic. He suffers with his plague-ridden patients but does not experience the illness himself, nor does he become a patient at any point. Nevertheless, he can feel empathy as he watches his patients suffer and die from plague. A good man and a competent physician, Dr. Rieux chronicles the events during the plague outbreak, for the most part in sober and factual language. However, when witnessing an innocent child's death from the plague, Dr. Rieux's style clearly shows his empathy. Contemplating the dying boy's agony, Dr. Rieux describes it metaphorically:

> And just then the boy had a sudden spasm, as if something had bitten him in the stomach, and uttered a long, shrill wail. For moments that seemed endless he stayed in a queer, contorted position, his body racked by convulsive tremors; it was as if his frail frame were bending before the fierce breath of the plague, breaking under the reiterated gusts of fever. Then the storm-wind passed, there came a lull, and he relaxed a little; the fever seemed to recede, leaving him gasping for breath on a dank, pestilential shore, lost in a languor that already looked like death. When for the third time the fiery wave broke on him, lifting him a little, the child curled himself up and shrank away to the edge of the bed, as if in terror of the flames advancing on him, licking his limbs. A moment later, after tossing his head wildly to and fro, he flung off the blanket. From between the inflamed eyelids big tears welled up and trickled down the sunken, leaden-hued cheeks. When the spasm had passed, utterly exhausted, tensing his thin legs and arms, on which, within forty-eight hours, the flesh had wasted to the bone, the child lay flat, racked on the tumbled bed, in a grotesque parody of crucifixion. (*The Plague*, 199)

Dr. Rieux's images show that his heart and imagination have been activated by watching the child die.

Dr. Rieux's language shows his empathy, but he needs no instruction in empathy, as he is naturally sensitive to others; the child's death stirs his feelings that were there all along. Dr. Rieux's own life has been difficult, but he has remained observant and respectful of others. During the plague epidemic, Dr. Rieux pities his patients, but he restrains his feelings (*The Plague*, 84, 86). With the plague deaths continuing, too much feeling for his patients may hinder him in his job as a physician. In an extreme situation such as the one Camus describes, the physician finds it necessary to "harden his heart protectively" (*The Plague*, 178). Occasionally, however, the good doctor's natural empathy erupts in his actions. The most notable example is Dr. Rieux's bursting into tears when his patient and friend Tarrou dies of the plague (*The Plague*, 269). Through the *persona* of Dr. Rieux, Camus has shown two things about empathy in a medical setting: the good physician usually feels empathy, but he knows how to limit its manifestations. Dr. Rieux tries to balance natural feeling with necessary reason.

Camus's novel analyzes empathy. He chooses as his hero an empathetic doctor. Fighting against overwhelming physical and metaphysical evil, this doctor tries to come to the aid of suffering humanity. If he had not shown natural empathy for people dying of the plague, Dr. Rieux would have been less likable. With his feelings under control, he can serve his patients effectively. Camus's fictional character makes an excellent role model for a balanced medical professional. He is connected to others yet fully intact and functioning.

The last example of natural empathy from literature occurs in *Winter's Child*, a series of stories about a group of patients waiting to give birth in a high-risk pregnancy ward in a Danish hospital. The hospital is the setting for these stories of childbirth with complications. Midwifery students, midwives, nurses, and doctors all work in the ward. Some are more sensitive to patients than others. One particular physician shows natural empathy, when he meets with a patient who has given birth to a little boy with no feet. The physician tries to tell the patient, Tenna, what has happened, but she will not hear. The doctor repeats the bad news:

> She is icy cold. He's wrong. He's not talking to her—it must be someone else.
>
> She hears him repeat everything all over again. The boy was apparently dead, but they have managed to bring him back to life. He weighs 1800 grams, but would probably have weighed a few hundred grams more if he had any feet.
>
> A group of specialists are at that moment examining him in the pediatric department.
>
> "What can I do?" says the doctor in despair. "It's not my fault." No,

naturally it's not his fault. He walks up and down the room, trying to get her to understand what has happened.

"Will he have to live in a wheelchair all his life?" says Tenna.

"I don't really know much about that," he says. "But it is immensely important that the boy has his knee-joints." (Moerch 1986, 144)

The doctor's despair at this tragedy, "It's not my fault," is perhaps not an extraordinary reaction. Dr. Ragin disclaimed responsibility for his patients' pain. Dr. Rieux sheds "tears of impotence," when his patient Tarrou dies (*The Plague*, 269). With this level of natural empathy there sometimes comes a recognition of individual, human powerlessness in the face of unconquerable evil. Suffering will never end. But since the naturally empathetic helper is interested in others as equals, he can find the courage to persevere despite constant defeat. In this case, empathy, or projecting one's own personality into the situation of another, can entail frustration with one's own limitations. Yet, as Camus's and Moerch's physicians show, one can choose to persevere.

Natural empathy can also lead to a fresh assessment of our own lives. Edith Stein has summarized this ego-directed benefit of empathy:

> By empathy with differently composed personal structures we become clear on what we are not, what we are more or less than others. Thus, together with self knowledge, we also have an important aid to self evaluation. Since the experience of value is basic to our own value, at the same time as new values are acquired by empathy, our own unfamiliar values become visible. When we empathically run into ranges of value locked to us, we become conscious of our own deficiency or disvalue. Every grasping of different persons can become the basis of a value comparison. Since, in the act of preference or disregard, values often come to givenness that remain unnoticed in themselves, we learn to assess ourselves correctly now and then. We learn to see that we experience ourselves as having more or less value in comparison with others. (Stein 1970, 105–6)

For most people, such self-assessment is a lifelong activity. If we notice our ability to learn, to feel, and to show empathy, perhaps we will give ourselves a higher assessment. Self-esteem may be enlarged. Empathy with the other may be good for ourselves.

Because literature and art appeal to valuable emotions, such as empathy, they need to be included in the education of young people whether they be future physicians or future patients or both. A humanistic approach to medicine puts the human being at the center. A faithful study of literature and art and medicine can link two cultures and two individuals. In addition, empathy is a part of the art of medicine and can probably be learned just as the scientific aspects of medicine can. The cultivation of empathy is a good thing for humans and especially for physicians. Finally, an appropriate balance, between reason and feeling and between concern with self and concern with others, can nurture in health care professionals a richer connectedness to all humanity.

Examples of empathetic lessons can also be derived from specific works of visual art that contain medical themes. In such works, the depiction of illness and suffering effectively communicates the physical and emotional sensations being experienced. The sensations that accompany illness, for example, nausea, pain, asthenia, are known by every human being from earliest childhood. This experience of illness leaves each of us with a distinct and often bitter memory of what being sick means. Visual artists have often drawn on their own experience of illness to create works of art. Indeed, sickness is one of the commonest themes found in art. For example, in current popular films, one finds excellent illustrations of the experience of illness.[1]

In previous epochs, illness represented an even greater threat to individual survival than it does today. Thus, it is not surprising that many works of visual art depict birth, illness, and death.[2]

James Gillray (1757–1815), an English caricaturist and illustrator, was at his best when lampooning various figures at the court of George III, known to Americans as the king who opposed the American Revolution. Gillray was a self-taught artist, although he did study both at the Royal Academy in London and on the Continent. During his life, he produced more than twelve thousand drawings and illustrations. His depiction of gout is typical of his work: exaggerated, if not grotesque. The agony of podagra is almost palpable in his illustration of the "gouty monster" sinking his claws and teeth into the ample flesh of his victim's forefoot.

Honoré Daumier (1808–1879) was the son of a Marseilles glazier who came to Paris with his family in 1816 at the age of eight. He studied with some of the best-known artists of his time but rapidly left off painting in the Salon style in order to create satiric characterizations of the bourgeoisie and the court of the emperor, Louis Phillippe. A particularly biting cartoon of the emperor led to six months' incarceration for Daumier. Lawyers, doctors, and politicians all felt the sharp edge of Daumier's wit. During his life, he created almost four thousand

1. *Camille Claudel, Whose Life Is It Anyway?, One Flew over the Cuckoo's Nest, Coming Home, The Elephant Man*, and *Judgement at Nuremberg* are some recent films on medical topics.

2. Birth: see illustrations to D. T. Moerch, *Winter's Child*; illness: Albrecht Dürer, *Melencolia, I*, 1514 (Fogg Museum of Art, Harvard University, Cambridge, Mass.); death: Jacques-Louis David, *The Death of Socrates*, 1787 (Metropolitan Museum of Art, New York).

drawings and lithographs. Daumier's depiction of physicians often focuses on their greed, showing doctors asking for excessive fees from helpless patients. A lithograph by Daumier reveals the agony of a severe headache. Similar dramatizations have been used in contemporary advertisements for headache remedies. One wonders if Daumier himself suffered from migraine headaches, so immediate and convincing is the depiction of the headache sufferer.

Alfred Rethel (1816–1859) was a German historical painter and draftsman. Most of his short career was spent painting with oils on canvases and on walls. He created a famous fresco on the wall of the town hall at Aachen depicting scenes from the life of Charlemagne. A famous wood engraving by Rethel is entitled *The Dance of Death*. It is both emotional and precise, reminding one of the dissolution of human society during epidemic and war. Death the Destroyer is shown riding toward a besieged town. This engraving is from the series *Another Dance of Death* (1849), which depicts events from the revolutions of 1848. The imaginative depiction of the traditional dance of death is reminiscent of Edgar Allan Poe's short story "The Mask of the Red Death," in which a deadly epidemic strikes down revelers at a masked ball.

The message that emanates from these three selected works of art is clear: illness and death can strike one at any time. The artist reminds his viewers that pain and suffering are an everyday human occurrence. No one is immune. Through bad fortune, the king can soon enough become the fool; in an instant, the doctor can find himself in the patient's place.

References

Camus, A. 1972. *The Plague*. Trans. S. Gilbert. New York: Random House.

Chekhov, A. 1974. *Ward Number Six and Other Stories*. Trans. R. Hingley. New York: Oxford University Press.

Liddell, H. G., and R. Scott. 1966. *A Greek-English Lexicon*. Oxford: Clarendon Press.

Moerch, D. T. 1986. *Winter's Child*. Trans. Joan Tate. Lincoln: University of Nebraska Press.

Montaigne, M. de. 1973. "On the education of children." In *Selections from the Essays*, ed. and trans. D. M. Frame. Arlington Heights, Ill.: AHM Publishing.

Shakespeare, W. 1963. *The Tragedy of King Lear*. Ed. R. Fraser. New York: New American Library.

Snow, C. P. 1981. *The Two Cultures and a Second Look*. Cambridge: Cambridge University Press.

Stein, E. 1970. *On the Problem of Empathy*. Trans. W. Stein. The Hague: Martinus Nijhoff.

Williams, W. C. 1967. *The Autobiography*. New York: New Directions.

Chapter 14
The Narrative Road
to Empathy

R I T A   C H A R O N

Three patients presented me with problems of interpretation and meaningfulness. These were my medical chart notes early in our work together:

Case 1: R.F. is a twenty-two-year-old woman born in the Dominican Republic and now living in Yonkers who has a history of migraine headaches and chronic low back pain unrelated to trauma or skeletal abnormality. She has never been hospitalized for either condition. She has been intermittently treated with Fioricet for the migraine headaches and nonsteroidal anti-inflammatory agents for the back pain with some relief of symptoms. She presents to the office, without an appointment, to ask that the physician sign her disability forms.

Case 2: H.B. is a sixty-eight-year-old woman with hypertension, non–insulin-dependent diabetes mellitus, coronary artery disease, degenerative joint disease, and paroxysmal supraventricular tachycardia well controlled on Verapamil. She presents acutely with a three-day history of nonproductive cough, low-grade fever, and myalgias. She received her influenza vaccination this fall. On physical examination, she is afebrile and the chest is clear. The patient insists on having a chest X-ray despite assurance that there is no evidence of pneumonia. On further questioning, she reports that a neighbor in her apartment building has been recently documented to have pulmonary tuberculosis.

Case 3: An eighty-four-year-old man with lung cancer metastatic to the brain and liver is admitted to the medical service in August for pain control and terminal care. His family has come to New York from the South to be with him as he dies. The medical intern attempts aggressive fluid management and wants to institute heroic intervention.

Although unremarkable to the doctor seeking pathophysiological challenge, these cases become interesting for the emotions they arouse: impatience, irritation, the feeling of being manipulated, helplessness, and uncertainty. The cases raise complex management problems—not whether to sign a disability form for a healthy person, not how to resist a patient's willful insistence on an inappropriate diagnostic test, and not setting treatment goals for patients with terminal illnesses—but how to solve problems of meaning in clinical work. In these ordinary cases and the legion like them, the doctor is called on to do the cognitive and affective work that will, through empathic connection with the patient, reveal the meaningfulness of the troubling behaviors of patients, of students, or of colleagues. What can help the doctor to find meaning in the lives of these relative strangers?

It is a commonplace in medicine that patients (and doctors) are to be treated like whole persons. Francis Peabody's injunction that "the secret of the care of the patient is in caring for the patient" graces many a textbook of medicine or guide to medical interviewing (Peabody [1927] 1984, 818). Exhortation and injunction fall short, however, of defining the skills doctors should be developing and the means by which they can develop them. Quick to do anything that will increase the effectiveness of their clinical actions, doctors need only be told how to increase their skills in the domains of empathy—not in ill-defined global normative but in programmatic and measurable terms—in order to try to master yet another realm of competence.

Narrative Knowledge and Logico-Scientific Knowledge

The competence one exercises in understanding the inappropriate request for a disability form or a chest X-ray resides in the domain of narrative knowledge. Irreducible to one another and both essential for effective medical practice, narrative knowledge and logico-scientific knowledge together allow humans to gather and to comprehend information about the world (Bruner 1986). Logico-scientific knowledge is used to collect and evaluate replicable, universal, generalizable, and empirically verifiable information. Driven by principled hypotheses and generated by so-called detached observers, logico-scientific knowledge relies on such formal operations as conjunction and dis-junction to establish testable propositions about general causes. The tools of such knowledge are mathematics, logic, and the sciences; its language must be nonallusive, nonambiguous, and reliable. By no means without creativity, this type of knowledge exercises the imagination in "seeing" a solution to a problem before it can be formally proven.

Narrative knowledge, on the other hand, concerns the motivations and the consequences of human actions. Always particularized, narrative knowledge seeks to examine and comprehend singular events, contextualized within their time and place. Newspaper stories, myths, fairy tales, novels, Scripture, and clinical case histories are narratives: they all recount and interpret events, bound in some form of chronology, that have befallen humans or human surrogates. They all bear the stamp of their tellers, who are not detached observers but who actively participate in generating the stories they tell. They rely on such fea-tures as metaphor and allusion to convey messages about the particular and to suggest causal connections among random events. Narrative language reso-nates with multiple contradictory meanings, alludes to stories already told, and reveals affective as well as cognitive dimensions of the teller and the subjects. If logico-scientific knowledge is used to establish universally true features of the world by transcending the particular, narrative knowledge is used to reveal the particular and, in turn, to hint at universal truths. Through narrative knowl-edge, humans come to recognize themselves and each other, telling stories in order to know who they are, where they are from, and where they are going.

Doctors use both forms of knowledge in the laboratory and in the care of individual patients. In my earlier evaluation of H.B., for instance, I had assigned a tentative etiology to her cardiac arrhythmia based on what is known about the conduction system of the heart—any human heart—information that had been gathered through logico-scientific investigation. I had relied on the results of a Holter monitor, an echocardiogram, and a stress-thallium exam to test my hypotheses. To evaluate the results of these diagnostic tests, I had to consider their statistical predictive values and their relevance to the clinical questions I was asking. I had then to consider confounding factors that may have altered the reliability of these tests in this particular patient: gender, medications, or con-current diseases, for example, can alter the predictive value of many tests. Finally, I had to decide how to integrate these findings into the care of the patient: would she be able to institute behavior changes? Would her diabetes preclude use of a beta-blocker? Would she be able to afford a long-acting calcium-channel blocker? Finally, I instituted treatment in accord with these conclusions and evaluated her response to medical intervention, thereby accu-mulating more information regarding the possible causes and clinical features of her arrhythmia. A combination of both forms of knowledge, then, is used to perform clinical work—not one first and then the other, but a weaving of these mental processes by which a clinician applies what is known about the human body in general to the particular human body in question.[1]

Well trained in the logico-scientific method, doctors have until recently paid little attention to their narrative training. Yet, when one inspects the work of the clinician, one finds that the work of medicine in considerable part rests on the doctor's ability to listen to the stories patients tell, to make sense of these often chaotic accounts of illness, to inspect and evaluate the listener's personal response to the story being told, to understand what these narratives mean at multiple and sometimes contradictory levels, and to be moved by them. Clinical medicine emerges as an activity rooted in the particular, the casuistic, the longitudinal appreciation of meaning in the lives of others, an activity not dissimilar from reading fiction or interpreting the Scripture. Clearly, such activities as understanding motives and helping patients to make ethical decisions reside in the narrative domain; many clinicians are less aware that their narrative knowledge also allows them to perform such routine tasks as taking a medical history, interpreting a physical finding, reaching diagnoses, and teaching patients about what ails them.

Only with narrative competence can a physician deliver empathic care. Without the patient's robust narrative world the physician cannot enter into the patient's suffering world, cannot offer comfort, and cannot accompany the patient through the illness experience. Only doctors who have developed narrative competence will recognize their patients' motives and desires, will allow patients to tell their full stories of illness, and will offer themselves as therapeutic instruments.

We know what happens in the face of narrative incompetence. We get the story wrong. I concluded that the twenty-two-year-old woman with back pain was lazy and did not want to work. What else would explain her request for disability? Only because I was harried on the day she came in did I sign her disability form.

Being groomed as I am to deliver managed care, I refused to order a chest X-ray for Mrs. H.B. Instead, I ordered a cough suppressant, acetaminophen, and fluids. In view of her neighbor's tuberculosis, I arranged for the appropriate skin test to be planted.

When the intern precipitated pulmonary edema by aggressively hydrating

---

1. Some argue that narrative knowledge underlies not only the care of individual patients but also the generation and trustworthiness of theoretical constructs that explain physiological and pathophysiological processes (Hunter 1991).

the patient with lung cancer, I insisted that he follow strict guidelines for so-called comfort measures. No blood tests, no X-rays, no antibiotics—only pain control and skin medicines.

In all three cases, my initial management was narratively incompetent. I did not understand the meanings of the unruly behavior I was attempting to address. I left the office and the ward feeling stingy and ineffective. More saliently, I knew that the patients and the intern probably felt unheard or demeaned by my behavior and that my interventions, rather than having been therapeutic or educational, had been punitive. In part, the irritation and anxiety doctors experience is caused by such lapses in narrative competence. Harry Stack Sullivan reminds us that the effective interview, psychiatric or otherwise, allows the person interviewed to feel better at the end of it than at the beginning (Sullivan 1970). It may also be true that the effective interaction allows the interviewer to feel satisfied, generous, and at peace. Feelings of irritation and anxiety, then, may be signs of the doctor's ineffectiveness in narrative domains.

Improving Narrative Competence

How can doctors improve their narrative competence? Exercise in narrative competence would help doctors to (1) recognize the complex and contradictory narratives of illness; (2) increase the accuracy of their observations and interpretation of physical signs, behavior, and emotional concerns; (3) be moved by the stories of suffering; (4) make themselves available to accompany patients through their troubles; and (5) as a bonus, more fully allow meaning into their own lives. Let me suggest three methods for increasing narrative competence and therefore the capacity for empathy. The first is to write; the second is to read; the third is to recognize the ways in which medicine strikes home.

WRITING I wrote a story about the young woman from Yonkers with back pain. Feeling guilty later for not having taking the time to hear her out and confused about both her behavior and my response, I made up a set of circumstances that gave her a motive: in my fantasy, she wanted to work as a model and needed to support a move to Manhattan while she prepared a portfolio and went to auditions. I was her last hope, for she had already been turned down for several jobs and she knew no one who could lend her money. Written from the patient's point of view, the story showed that the patient felt demeaned by my brusque treatment of her, that the signature on the disability form was hardly worth the abrupt dismissal.

When I next saw the patient, I found myself much more solidly on her side, having spent time imagining her perspective. Because of this new alliance, I was able to question her much more fully about her circumstances, discovering that much of what I had imagined was true. Lean and muscular, the clinical imagination knows more than one consciously knows. Writing allows access to that imaginative knowledge, and with it to empathic knowledge of the patient. Over time, I learned that I had been only half right. In fact, she did need the disability to allow her to move from her parents' home. She came to my office that day in desperation, but I had no idea how desperate she was. Gradually, she trusted me enough to tell of the physical and sexual abuse that she and her sisters suffered at the hands of their father. She had to set up a safe home in Manhattan for her sisters and herself. By now, I care for her mother and her sisters, and I continue to take care of her. Last month, she asked me to become her father's internist as well.

A fourth-year medical student asked me to help her write about a difficult clinical episode that occurred on her surgical rotation. An insightful and courageous woman, this student realized that a dramatic night on call with the transplant team had activated painful memories, had turned her against her medical colleagues, and had threatened her motivation for being a doctor. She wrote a compelling story about that night, including the memories and associations elicited by the events. Only by writing was the student able to recognize the full meaning of that night. Only when her feelings and sensations achieved the status of narrative language could she free herself from that night and acknowledge her own bravery. She knows herself more profoundly now, not only for the experience but for the telling of it.

READING Not everyone will feel ready to write imaginatively about patients or about themselves. Reading, however, is a skill all doctors bring with them to medical school. The most narrowly trained science major will have read some fiction, attended some plays, watched some movies, and imaginatively experienced the lives of others. Practitioners in the young field of literature and medicine have been teaching literature in medical schools and hospitals in order to increase students' capacity for empathy. Reading serious fiction exercises the narrative skills of adopting alien perspectives, of imagining moral landscapes, and of experiencing other lives as reality. In his "Defense of Poetry," which includes allusive and metaphoric prose as well as poems, Percy Shelley describes the imagination as "the great instrument of moral good . . . [that] strengthens that faculty which is the organ of the moral nature of man, in the same manner as exercise strengthens a limb" (Shelley 1930, 8:118). Shelley makes explicit the connections among the imagination, the moral good, and empathy: "A man, to be greatly good, must imagine intensely and comprehensively; he must put himself in the place of another . . . the pains and pleasures of his species must become his own" (Shelley 1930, 8:118).

By reading fiction, medical students and doctors can strengthen their ability to enter narrative worlds and to interpret them on that world's terms. A medical student reads Flaubert's "A Simple Heart." A poor peasant woman becomes increasingly impoverished: she is deceived by a young man she loves, a young child in her care dies of pneumonia, her beloved nephew dies at sea, and finally her parrot—companion to her world constricting through deafness and blindness—dies. Undaunted, she has the parrot stuffed and, by the end of her life, finds her eyes gently shifting from the picture of the Holy Ghost to the stuffed parrot during prayer. Is Felicité a simpleton, a psychotic, or a devout believer? How can a young man at the end of the twentieth century make sense of the actions of this mid-nineteenth-century peasant woman who prays to a stuffed parrot? Can he find methods of interpreting her actions so that they take on meaning? Is pity or laughter all he finds in his emotional response to her plight? A student can be encouraged to recognize Felicité's series of losses, her sequence of futile attachments, and her resigned yet defiant acceptance of her fate, glorified through her own insistence that it mean something. When this student takes care of a hospitalized homeless woman with AIDS, or of a middle-aged profoundly retarded man with pneumonia, or of a Cambodian survivor of Khmer Rouge atrocities, he will use these same skills of recognition and interpretation of strangers, joining these patients in the attempt to make sense out of chaos, pain, and loss. His recognition of his patients will not only allow him to comfort them; it will allow him to observe and accurately interpret their behavior, their complaints, their disease processes, and their response to treatment.

Is not literature, some ask, a detour away from clinical activity? Why not involve students in the lives of their patients rather than asking them to pretend that fictional characters are as important as live people? After quoting Goethe's *Wilhelm Meister* in *Civilization and Its Discontents*, Freud writes that it is "vouch-safed to a few to salvage without effort from the whirlpool of their own feelings the deepest truths, towards which the rest of us have to find our way through tormenting uncertainty and with restless groping" (Freud 1953–74, 21:133). Freud's few are, of course, literary artists. Flaubert was able to see and to tell Felicité's story through the agency of his art. His gifts granted him the ability to weave his own autobiography, the history of his nation, and the account of this farming village and its petty yet genuine inhabitants into a seamless narrative of memory and unbounded love. Only through the power of his artistic gift could

Flaubert have imagined this woman Felicité, to whom so much was denied and who yet remained resilient and radiant of faith, and to have comprehended and displayed the inner power of her simple heart.

In clinical work, both doctors and patients often experience the tormenting uncertainty and the restless groping that can find expression only through poetry. I had admitted an elderly woman with end-stage breast cancer to the hospital some time ago. The patient of my vacationing partner, this woman was a stranger to me. I knew more about her neuroanatomy than about her life. I knew, though, that she was soon to die, and my responsibility was to effect so-called placement: to transfer her to a hospice for terminal care. In my calendar book next to her Presbyterian Hospital unit number I copied a short section of William Carlos Williams's long poem "Asphodel, That Greeny Flower":

> It is difficult
> to get the news from poems
>   yet men die miserably every day
>   for lack
> of what is found there.
>   Hear me out
>   for I too am concerned
> and every man
>   who wants to die at peace in his bed
>   besides.
>   (Williams 1962, 161–62)

The poem helped to remind me of my task—yes, to check serial head computed tomography (CT) scans to determine the need for additional radiotherapy; yes, to maximize oxygenation and comfort through the judicious use of broncho-dilators and steroids; yes, to evaluate for treatable depression in the face of her realistic sadness. And, yes, to allow this elderly woman to talk about her life, to reach for those important to her, and to die at peace in her bed besides.

Reading makes one reach into the inner self. Although not at all medically specific, this outcome of reading can be a critical contributing factor to mature empathic clinical care. After reading Henry James's "The Beast in the Jungle," a medical student articulated her own sense of destiny. The protagonist in the story believes that something dramatic will happen to him. He spends most of his life waiting for the beast to lunge; in the end he realizes, with the help of a woman who loves him, that his fate was to have been "the man of his time, *the* man, to whom nothing on earth was to have happened . . . all the while he had waited the wait was itself his portion" (James 1908, 17:125). Daughter of a successful and now terminally ill physician, the student faced her own feelings of helplessness in the face of her and her father's destiny. Reading and discussing James helped her to recognize her wishes to be delivered of her urgent fate and to accept the pain (and potential joy) of caring for her parents through the ordeal of her father's illness. In the woman character in the story, the student found a model of empathic and activating caring, a model that helped her both to understand her father's work and to make sense of her own. Months later, after her father had died, she wrote an insightful essay about the James story, including her own journey of loss within her reflections on the short story.

Sometimes individual stories help in the care of individual patients. Internist Julie Connelly writes about the manner in which Tolstoy's "Death of Ivan Ilyich" helped her in caring for a particular dying patient (Connelly 1990). More commonly, the act of reading itself builds toward clinical and empathic competence. Paying close attention to language, diction, metaphor, and reader response in texts permits one to pay similarly close attention to the language, mode of speaking, metaphorical content, and allusiveness of patients' histories. Reading expands one's capacity to tolerate ambiguity, to live with uncertainty, and to read (or hear) stories to the end. (A corporeal hunger develops in the reader to read stories to the end or to read all the works of an author to the end. It is an insatiable and delirious joy.) The skilled reader is an ever-active reader. "Why is she telling me this now?" the reader will ask of her author. "Whose point of view is being recorded here?" "Why does this passage make me feel so sad?"

My skills of reading allowed me to understand Mrs. H.B. She floored me with her account of her neighbor with tuberculosis. Because it was unusual for this patient to be unreasonable, I found my curiosity mounting. Generally placid if not withdrawn, the patient was today quite distressed, a behavioral sign that required explanation. "Why is she doing this now?" I wondered. As I made out the order slip for the skin test, I asked her how her neighbor had gotten the disease: "Tell me about your neighbor with TB."

She told me that her seventy-five-year-old neighbor wanted a husband. She went up to Attica II, the state prison on the Hudson River, and got one. Three years ago, she married a thirty-eight-year-old prisoner. Assuring me that this was not atypical behavior for elderly single or widowed women in the city, my patient explained that the prisoner had AIDS at the time of the marriage and had since developed tuberculosis. He was released only a few weeks ago, his sentence perhaps shortened because of his illness and because he had a wife and a home waiting for him. He died three weeks after coming home to his wife. She caught his tuberculosis while nursing him that short time. Fortunately ("She says they used safe sex," my patient reported), the wife seems not to have contracted the HIV infection.

I knew the source of my patient's distress. I repeated my assurance that her lungs sounded fine and made sure she would return to have her skin test read. I explained to her the transmission patterns of the tubercle bacillus, relieving her anxiety that minimal casual contact with her neighbor at the mailboxes could have infected her. It was only after she had left the office, however, that I thought to ask the next narrative question, "Why did she tell me that whole story?" Was she thinking about getting a husband from Attica II? Was her own lonely withdrawn life diminished in contrast to the tragic but engaged life of her neighbor? I recognized personal judgmental feelings about elderly women who marry in such circumstances, ranging from disdain at the individuals seemingly so desperate for companionship to sad rage that women's status is so low that a convict with a terminal illness is considered a decent catch for a woman twice his age. However, if my patient were considering such an action, I would have to make sure that she understood the health risks and the means of protecting herself. Furthermore, I would have to do so without communicating the automatic derision of my initial response to the tale.

I had recently taught "A Simple Heart," and perhaps Felicité was on my mind. The actions of my patient's neighbor were not unlike Flaubert's peasant woman who forms inappropriate attachments in asymmetric love relationships. As I realized the similarity in emotional landscape between the two stories, I could think more clearly about the potential meaning of the neighbor's marriage. Certainly, my initial disdain caused me to explore the tangible benefits first. Must it not be that the partners in such a marriage gain insurance benefits or become eligible for Medicaid? A matter of convenience, no doubt, the marriage probably shortens the prisoner's sentence or grants the wife rights to a larger Section 8 apartment. And yet, like Felicité, might there not be a genuine human expression of need and love in the action?

This train of thought led to a consideration of my patient's place in the world. She lives alone. Her adult children have little to do with her. She had recently had a string of vexing problems with her landlord, with Con Edison (the local gas and electric vendor), and with the telephone company: all were trying to deny her services. No doubt she felt victimized and tenuous in her current barely adequate living situation. Perhaps a marriage of convenience would improve her material circumstances. As I ruminated, I realized that I knew of no one in her life save health professionals and characters in soap operas. The readerly question "Why is she telling me this now?" insisted on an answer. Was the story in fact about herself and not the surrogate neighbor? Next time I see her, I will find out more about her own plans and hopes for companionship and commitment and about the metaphorical connection between her friend and herself. This process of reading, ruminating, setting aside my own biases, and allowing for the possible meaningfulness of behavior I had been quick to judge accomplished the needed clinical task: it replaced my judgmental response with an empathic one. The clinical imagination never stops.

RECOGNIZING THAT MEDICINE STRIKES HOME He was a very good intern. Why was he still doing blood gases on this moribund elderly man? Remembering the hell of internship in August, I tried to imagine what could be prompting the intern to continue the inappropriate care. On a hunch, I asked him if anyone in his family had been sick recently. His grandfather had died just that spring. Yes, he had died of lung cancer. Once he said it, and only then, could my intern see what he was doing. He was trying to save the life of his grandfather's surrogate, doing for this stranger what he felt guilty for not having done for his grandfather. As soon as we spoke, he stopped the inappropriate care, joined the family grieving around the patient's bedside, and helped the man to die without pain. No doubt his death allowed him to mourn his own grandfather more fully as well.

Because they recount individual lives and culminate with their deaths, medical narratives may well be considered un-narratives, that is, pure generative sources to narratives that follow. "All narrative may be in essence obituary," suggests literary critic Peter Brooks, "in that . . . the retrospective knowledge that it seeks . . . stands on the far side of the end, in human terms on the far side of death" (Brooks 1985, 95). We humans seek the knowledge that exists beyond death—the knowledge, that is, of death's meaning and consequences—and we doctors, as specialized agents licensed to know more than others about death's domain, bear great responsibility toward our knowledge. How little we realize others hunger for what we come to know as a matter of course. One proof of such hunger is to be found in fiction, as critic Walter Benjamin observes: "The meaning of the character's life is revealed only in his death. . . . What draws the reader to the novel is the hope of warming his shivering life with a death he reads about" (Benjamin 1969, 100–101).[2] By virtue of our work, then, we doctors have an opportunity to be deeply learned in the ways of life. Despite the painfulness of closeness to death, as my intern discovered in August, we are granted the great privilege of drawing close to death, of giving others comfort from what we have learned about it, and of warming our lives with the meaningfulness that shows only as life ends.

My intern's experience documented the intimately personal power of medi-

2. Literary critics concerned with such elements of literature as plot and narrative structure and theory are particularly helpful to doctors who are trying to understand the narrative elements in their clinical work (Booth 1983; Mitchell 1981; and Martin 1986).

cal practice. Second-year medical students are stunned to realize how painful a medical relationship can be. "What happens," a student asked in a medical interviewing seminar, "if the patient's problem is something that you are personally having to deal with? What happens if it strikes home?" At age twelve, this student had lost her mother to gastric cancer, and she had just interviewed a patient whose mother had been diagnosed with the same disease. I had to explain gently that much of medicine, if practiced effectively, strikes home. We doctors can get personally injured by our patients, developing drug-resistant TB or hepatitis or AIDS from contact with our patients. We also can get emotionally and existentially wounded by patients who arouse anxieties or who, through transference and countertransference, force us to reexperience painful episodes in our own lives or to face unresolved ongoing conflicts. As we get more skilled in our work, we learn not to dodge reminders of personal suffering, but to allow our own injuries to increase the potency of our care of patients, to allow our personal experiences to strengthen the empathic bond with others who suffer.

Coda

"The secret of the care of the patient is in caring for the patient." What is the secret of caring for the patient? Caring for the patient—or empathy—can be understood, exercised, strengthened, and enjoyed through reclaiming narrative knowledge. Underexposed to narrative knowledge and overschooled in the logico-scientific, doctors gradually lose their abilities to tell and to be moved by stories of human suffering unless they actively and courageously replenish their stores of imaginative vision, unless they recall how to get the news from a poem. Not superficially but deeply and with great accuracy must doctors grasp, see, contain, reflect, recognize until they can *tell* the full and painful stories that befall their patients and themselves. Then will they have ears to hear, then will they have the capacity to tolerate their patients' pain and to extend through empathy their deep and lasting help. As Henry James says of the reader, the doctor's task is "to lend himself, to project himself and steep himself, to feel and feel till he understands and to understand so well that he can say" (James 1981, 136). Therein lies the task, therein the gift and gladness.

References

Benjamin, W. 1969. *Illuminations: Essays and Reflections.* Trans. H. Zohn. New York: Schocken Books.

Booth, W. 1983. *The Rhetoric of Fiction.* 2d ed. Chicago: University of Chicago Press.

Brooks, P. 1985. *Reading for the Plot: Design and Intention in Narrative.* New York: Random House.

Bruner, J. 1986. *Actual Minds, Possible Worlds.* Cambridge: Harvard University Press.

Connelly, J. 1990. The whole story. *Literature and Medicine.* 9:150–61.

Freud, S. 1953–74. Civilization and its discontents. In *The Standard Edition of the Complete Psychological Works of Sigmund Freud,* ed. and trans. J. Strachey, vol. 21. London: Hogarth Press.

Hunter, K. M. 1991. *Doctors' Stories: The Narrative Structure of Medical Knowledge.* Princeton: Princeton University Press.

James, H. 1908. The beast in the jungle. In *The Novels and Tales of Henry James: The New York Edition,* vol. 17. New York: Charles Scribner's Sons.

James, H. 1981. *Selected Literary Criticism.* Ed. M. Shapira. Cambridge, England: Cambridge University Press.

Martin, W. 1986. *Recent Theories of Narrative.* Ithaca: Cornell University Press.

Mitchell, W. J. T., ed. 1981. *On Narrative.* Chicago: University of Chicago Press.

Peabody, F. W. [1927] 1984. The care of the patient. *Journal of the American Medical Association.* [88:877–82] 252:813–18.

Shelley, P. B. 1930. A defense of poetry. In *The Complete Works of Percy Bysshe Shelley,* ed. R. Ingpen and W. E. Peck, vol. 8. London: The Julian Editions.

Sullivan, H. S. 1970. *The Psychiatric Interview.* New York: W. W. Norton.

Williams, W. C. 1962. *Pictures from Bruegel and Other Poems.* New York: New Directions Books.

Chapter 15
Empathy: Using Resonance
Emotions in the Service
of Curiosity

JODI HALPERN

I am called to see Mr. L because the staff in the intensive care unit are worried about his will to live. A sudden, severe neurologic disorder has paralyzed him and left him partially dependent on a ventilator, with a tracheostomy. He is only now learning to speak through a tube, and due to muscle weakness, this requires a great deal of effort. Interns, residents, attendants, and nurses care for him. His present resident tells me that he is an enigma and cannot or will not answer their questions about depression and suicide. When I meet him, I see a helpless, locked-in, cachectic man, but one who is looking at the door with some interest to meet the psychiatrist. I greet him warmly, and I later realize, sorrowfully. His eyes glaze over, and he goes a million miles away. I see the apathy that worries the medical intensive care unit (MICU) staff. Gently I ask him if he can try to talk with me, and he struggles to speak a few words, trembling and red-faced. His wife and the MICU nurse show their sorrow in covert glances. In one or two minutes he begs to rest, and I feel ashamed for having pushed him to make this futile effort.

Later, I talk to his family and learn that he is the patriarch of a family of women, with three grown daughters and a wife who have always counted on him to be in control. They tell me of his business and athletic prowess, and their sense of hopelessness about what a life of inactivity would mean for him. I also learn that he had requested an older, male psychiatrist. With mixed feelings of concern and relief I ask my service chief if the patient should see a psychiatrist who meets that description (I am a young woman), but the service chief encourages me to try again.

I feel trepidation about meeting Mr. L again, but also curious about what *his* hopelessness about talking to me and *mine* about connecting with him are showing me about his situation. I imagine what it would be like to be a powerful older man, suddenly enfeebled, handled by one young doctor after the next, and now seeking help from a young woman about "my" daughter's age. I find myself moved to feel shame and rage at being trapped in a body that is weak and dependent. In light of this, I reenter his room and look him firmly in the eyes, and speak in a robust voice that is more suited to a business interaction than to comforting someone who is hurt. I ask with curiosity, "What is it about talking with me that you don't like?" He does not look at me but begins to tell me how angry he feels at the doctors, including me, for invading his privacy at all hours of the day and night to adjust his respirator and ask the same stupid questions, all for nothing. And he adds that seeing how much this upsets his wife only makes it worse. His words cause me to imagine, with a visceral sinking feeling of dread, that I am trapped in a dead body—"I" cannot even roll away—but yet I remain a physical specimen, the machine pumping my lungs. And I am splayed before "my" family. Moved by these images, I remain silent as he reprimands all of his doctors through me. After he pauses for a long while, I say how unspeakably horrible it is that this should have happened to him. He looks directly at me, and I see how sad his eyes are, as we begin our work together.

In this chapter I argue that clinical empathy is a unique form of understanding patients that requires physicians to be emotionally engaged yet also promotes the objectivity that their roles demand. In the first half of this chapter, I argue against the popular notion that empathy is purely cognitive and does not require that the physician actually feel something about the patient's situation. Physicians strive to detach themselves emotionally from patients in order to be objective, reliable practitioners. Resonating with the patient emotionally, however, plays an essential role in informing the physician about the patient's experience, even if it seemingly presents an additional burden to physicians. In the second half of this chapter, I argue that since the aim of *clinical* empathy is to understand the patient's distinct experience, emotional resonance is only a first step. Physicians must also be guided by curiosity that decenters them from their own reactions and their own presuppositions about patients.

The *Oxford English Dictionary* defines empathy as "the power of projecting one's personality into (and so fully comprehending) the object of contemplation." These are the words of Theodor Lipps, who is credited with first using the concept *Einfühlung* (translated as empathy) in 1903 (Hunsdahl 1967). Lipps was as interested in aesthetics as in psychology and had in mind a process of "feeling into" another person's experience on the model of being transported into a piece of music. His emphasis is on projecting one's *own* personality *into* a work of art or another person, rather than merely observing the work's form or the person's behavior externally.

However, given that physicians' primary goal is healing *other* people, many of them see cultivating empathy as akin to enjoying works of art about doctoring—appreciating the expression of their own humanity in others seems edifying, but inessential to the practice of medicine. This view arises in part because Lipps's emphasis is not quite right for *clinical* empathy. The goal of clinical empathy is to understand in a detailed, experiential way what the patient is feeling.

But why invoke the concept of empathy at all? That is, does practicing good medicine require that patients be understood experientially? Physicians agree that being able to effectively treat patients depends upon diagnosis. To diagnose means to distinguish between what is and what is not significant for the patient's illness. The source of this information is the patient's history, literally a story about the patient's illness (Judith Ross, pers. comm. with author), as well as the patient's physical presentation. Physicians need empathy to help patients tell their histories.

The role of empathy in eliciting information is threefold. First, by understanding the way the patients feel about the information given or withheld, physicians can time their questions and modulate their tone in a way that will invite rather than discourage communication. For example, my awareness of Mr. L's shame influenced the way I asked him for his story. Second, given that diagnoses rely on symptoms, empathy contributes directly to diagnosis by enabling physicians to grasp the particular subjective complaints of the patients. For example, to distinguish between causes of a month of lethargy ranging from anemia to depression, it is important to know exactly why the discouraged patient stopped doing anything. Did she stop trying to be active after seeing she repeatedly had no energy for doing the things she wanted to do, or did she just stop wanting to do anything right from the start? Third, empathy plays an essential role in grasping the health values of patients and their families in order to make a treatment plan that can actually be adhered to. For example, in the case of Mr. L, it seemed he had become despondent and was increasingly refusing all treatment. Yet by understanding precisely what his goals were, and their complex effect on his family, I could assist him along the path toward rehabilitation.

Empathy Requires Emotional Engagement

But even if empathy is acknowledged as valuable for medical practice, physicians see it as problematic. In particular, the idea that they need to actually be moved by patients to provide good care seems to threaten their own ideal concerning their conduct towards patients—the ideal of "detached concern." "Detached concern" is an intent to heal or help patients that is independent of the physician's own emotional responses to patients. Physicians see their emotions as projections of their own needs or wishes onto patients that interfere with making objective diagnoses and providing reliable care.

The goal of detaching emotionally in order to be an objective observer of human nature has accompanied the rise of scientific medicine in the twentieth century. Physicians see how scientific data has contributed to their efficacy, and hence have eagerly taken on the mantle of the scientist for all aspects of their conduct. Codes of medical ethics identify *practicing* medicine "scientifically" (Beauchamp and Childress 1979) as an overarching ideal.[1] To gather data about patients that is "scientific," physicians prefer observations that are independent of their personalities, that others can reliably observe and measure—for example, radiologic studies and chemical assays. Yet the ideal of grounding medicine in scientific data is not sufficient for supporting the ideal of emotional detachment for medical practice.[2]

An additional reason that physicians detach themselves is that they see emotional involvement with the suffering of patients as too burdensome given the limitations on their time and energy. Physicians today often care for strangers in bureaucracies that demand that they maximize their efficiency by spending minimal time with patients. In addition, they must work long hours to master the expanding science and technology of medicine that make it possible to treat disease much more effectively than ever before. Physicians avoid feelings because they cannot take on the suffering of so many patients without having the time to grieve, or (when they are on call) even to sleep or see their own loved

1. "A physician should practice a method of healing founded on a scientific basis; and he should not voluntarily associate professionally with anyone who violates this principle" (T. Beauchamp and J. Childress. 1979. AMA Code of Ethics. In *Principles of Biomedical Ethics*. New York: Oxford University Press).

2. Some scientific evidence for the efficacy of a good emotional bond between physician and patient is considered in Spiro 1986.

one. Providing reliable care for one patient after the next in settings that resemble assembly lines in their anonymity and compartmentalization, physicians strive to make themselves into reliable instruments for treating disease. Yet physicians still have the goal of understanding and caring for their patients as human beings. The ideal of "detached concern" represents the hope that the goals of objectivity, reliability, and caring for patients are all compatible.

This hopefulness shows in several articles from the early 1960s that narrowly predate the medical ethics movement of the past three decades with its emphasis on the failure of physician-patient communication. In their 1963 essay on "Training for 'Detached Concern,'" Rene Fox and Howard Lief claim that by becoming detached, physicians also become better at understanding patients *empathically*. They describe advanced medical students as better at empathic listening because they are able to suppress their own emotions in the face of the patient's suffering in the same way they learned to suppress their personal responses to dissecting a cadaver (Fox and Lief 1963, 12–35).

Classic articles on "Sympathy and Empathy" (Aring 1958, 167:4) and on "Caring for the Patient" (Blumgart 1964, 270:9) also argue that physicians can be both emotionally detached and empathic. The two physicians argue that empathy is entirely intellectual in contrast to sympathy, in which physicians are moved by their patients. By sympathy these authors do not mean pity (which may involve little understanding of another and is easily distinguishable from empathy). Rather, they define sympathy broadly in terms that are akin to Lipps's definition of empathy: "The act or capacity of entering into or sharing the feelings of another." In contrast to sympathy, Aring describes empathy as making inferences about the patient's conditions from one's prior knowledge of emotions. Blumgart conceives of "neutral empathy" as the careful observation of the habits and attitudes of patients so that one can predict their responses to illness.

In arguing against these papers, I want first to acknowledge an important distinction between empathy and sympathy that they bring out. Sympathy involves reactivity and advocacy. The sympathizer feels an immediate motivation to alleviate suffering. For example, in sympathy I felt the need to protect Mr. L from further intrusive interviews. In contrast, empathy does not necessarily involve a pull of this sort (Melvin Lansky, pers. comm. with author). In empathy, I was curious about Mr. L's feelings of being intruded on, rather than moved to react to them by refraining from interviewing him.

The point that empathy itself does not necessarily involve advocacy may disturb some readers, but it is akin to saying that surgery does not involve advocacy and points out the need for using all clinical skills in the context of promoting the patient's health. We might then say that *clinical* empathy should involve a healing intent toward the patient. The point is that empathy does not necessarily involve sharing the motives of the person whose feelings one is imagining. This is made clear by considering how empathy can even be used to harm another; for example, people make particularly pointed barbs in anger when they grasp empathically what makes the other person feel most vulnerable.

However, the fact that empathy does not necessarily involve advocacy does not imply that empathy is independent of emotional engagement. The observation that I was able to overcome my sympathetic aversion to intruding on Mr. L out of genuine curiosity about his experience does not mean that my curiosity was devoid of fellow feelings; in fact it was not. (And even the fact that empathy can be used to hurt another does not show that empathy is devoid of fellow feelings, since loving feelings themselves can be misused sadistically.)

The idea that empathy is purely cognitive arises from additional assumptions. Empathy is pictured as an ordinary form of inferential reasoning that simply has a special subject matter. The physician observes the patients' words and gestures and then taps her knowledge of what typical emotional experiences are like (perhaps relying on some of her own past experiences, or those of other patients), and then applies her knowledge to the patient inferentially, without actually feeling sympathetic emotions.

But even if the physician knows a great deal about human emotions, how could she use this to infer something *new* about the patient? The idea is that the empathizer uses her knowledge of emotions to make predictions about the patient's internal world. Medical knowledge often involves predictions about something unknown, for example, the future course of a disease, based on something present and observable, such as the patient's biological condition. The idea that empathy is just another type of detached reasoning is modeled on this picture of prediction in science. The empathizer is seen as a kind of weather forecaster, observing the patient's changing expressions and predicting the weather conditions as accurately as possible.

Let us think through this model of empathy as observation and prediction, since it captures part of the truth. Empathy does require *working* from something observable to something that is not observable through ordinary sense perception. And empathic understanding involves generating hypotheses in that physicians need to test their grasp of the patient's feelings and modify their views according to the patient's feedback. But the sense in which empathic understanding involves "rough drafts" that can be confirmed or rejected characterizes all knowledge: if knowledge could not be evaluated in some way, then it could not be meaningful in the first place. For example, it would be meaningless to say that someone knows how to folk dance if there were no criteria for confirming or rejecting this or that gesture as an instance of folk dancing. Such criteria make it possible for a folk dancer to learn by trial and error—making moves, and then seeing how they are off and correcting them. But knowing how to folk dance cannot be a matter of making predictions—imagine the awkwardness of a dancer who operates by predicting where her feet should go next. Hence the fact that empathic understanding must involve trial and error does not mean that empathy can be accurately characterized as making predictions.

Most important, the content one holds in mind *while empathizing* is not "factual" information about the patient's observable conditions, such as: "Mr. L is angry" or even "Mr. L is enraged at his family for pitying him." Rather, empathy is more like daydreaming—one imagines what it is like to be in an experience. In the encounter with Mr. L, my thoughts revolve around feeling trapped in a useless body and feeling furious at all these doctors and nurses for pushing "me" around with their agile limbs. If we continue with the weather analogy, the thought content of empathy is that of someone who is actually in the storm and thinking: look at that rain, it's going to be soaking wet here unless it stops soon. This experiential perspective differs from that of the weather forecaster estimating the probability of the rain stopping.

But how can empathizers imagine what it is like to experience another person's emotions, since they cannot step into the patient's world in the way they can literally join someone else in the rain? The experiential content of empathy comes from the listener's prereflective capacity to resonate emotionally with another person. By emotional resonance, I mean the spontaneous experience of emotion stimulated by another person's like emotion, without necessarily holding in mind what they see as joyful or fearful. This spreading of emotion prior to deliberate thought is sometimes referred to as "contagion" and is most dramatically displayed in the frenzy of a mob, but it also occurs when an anxious person makes one immediately anxious, or a joyful person lightens one's mood spontaneously.

The example of the frenzied mob should make it immediately apparent that resonance emotions are necessary, but not sufficient, for clinical empathy with its purpose of learning something new about the patient. Resonance emotions are like stage lighting that sets the mood for a play in that they provide an appropriate mental landscape for the listener to weave together the details of the protagonist's story into a whole.

Placing the patient's words and gestures into a proper emotional context is often essential for providing effective medical care. For example, I resonated with Mr. L's desperation at being infantilized by his caregivers, and took his barrage of complaints as an indication of how deep and pervasive his feelings of helplessness were. This guided me to help him set boundaries for when and how he would receive pulmonary and other treatments, increasing his feelings of independence and his adherence to his treatment. If in contrast, I heard his complaints as petulant rather than feeling the desperation behind them, I might have used the solicitous tones one uses with someone being grumpy. This would probably have contributed to his feelings of infantilization, alienating him further from critical medical treatment.

It is possible that even if I had felt nothing, I would still have been able to predict that this man would respond better to medical treatment if given more control over his care. But the shortcomings of relying on such predictions in the absence of resonance are threefold. First, physicians will miss crucial aspects of the patient's individual experience that are not features of the doctors' prior generalizations; and they will expect reactions that, while typical, may not be *this* person's reactions. Second, they will lack the capacity to *follow* the patient's own story experientially and thus lack practical knowledge about when and how to say or do the right thing. The physician would be like someone who goes to the theater only to note those aspects of the drama that correspond to what she reads in the program synopsis, but not to *experience* the story. They would have no clue about how to gasp, sigh, and cry appropriately with the audience. Third, the patient will most likely see this combination of being mistakenly stereotyped and being *alone* in her dramatic moments as signs of disinterest on the physicians' part and will be unlikely to feel sufficient trust to openly reveal her history and to gain the reassurance that has therapeutic benefit.

In summary, it is mistaken to picture empathy as just another way physicians make use of their capacity to make scientific inferences about the patient. Sawyier, a philosopher of science, notes that, "When we fill in the concept of empathy, part of what we imply is that the empathizer has himself had something happen to him right then; it is not just that he has thought hard, or tried to figure something out" (Sawyier 1974, 37–47). This leads us to reject the ideal of the detached thinker for empathy because it denies the two experiential poles of empathic understanding: in empathy one grasps, more or less, *how* the other person experiences her situation; and at the same time the empathizer herself *experiences* the other's attitudes as presences, rather than as mere possibilities.

Emotions Are Essential for Understanding Reality

In order to understand how the physician's resonance emotions contribute to empathic understanding and also what threat this poses to the goals of objectivity and reliability, let us consider what role emotions play in thinking in general.

Emotions are not mere bodily feelings, like twinges. Nor are emotions reducible to behavioral descriptions, even though there are typical behaviors that correspond to emotions, like running away in fear. What is essential to emotions is that they are always *about* something, whether it be something as focused as fear of a scary tiger or as unfocused as sadness about the futility of one's daily activities.

Emotions do pose a challenge for physicians, because their thought content is not "objective" in that we do not expect emotional portrayals to be free from the person's particular perspective. Rather, the person who is afraid of a dog may see the dog's bark as a threat, whereas a happy dog-lover may see the dog's bark as a vigorous greeting. And these portrayals require emphasizing certain aspects of reality over others, so that, for example, part of fearing the scary dog is not noticing the dog's friendliness, and vice versa.[3]

Given that emotions involve being moved personally in ways that lead one to emphasize some aspects of reality over others, they have often been conceived of as sources of irrationality. The idea is that what is real is what can be observed objectively, so that the dog's scariness or attractiveness—qualities that are not judicable by objective criteria—is illusory. The problem with this view is that most of what matters to human beings does not conform to objective descriptions.

A world devoid of such "subjective" information as the warmth or aloofness of other people, or the excitement of meeting a goal, would be a world devoid of vitality; yet these phenomena are palpated not with technological instruments but with one's own emotion-based attunement to reality. If we take the psychological lives of human beings to be real, then it is irrational to exclude emotions as a source of information about reality. All human activity presupposes an emotional orientation that carves out a relevant niche and makes organized thought possible. By this account, even the apparently detached scientist would have an emotion directing her attention—perhaps an outwardly focused emotion like curiosity, or perhaps a self-related emotion like pride.

The idea that emotions are necessary to determine human relevance (deSousa 1987) coheres with an argument for the importance of emotions in directing long-term pursuits as well as spontaneous attention. Emotions can tether our interest in activities for prolonged periods of time, enabling us to develop enduring skills and interests. For example, in order to imagine individuals persisting in the long and difficult process of becoming physicians, we need

3. This is not to deny the experience of ambivalence in which one has more than one emotion toward a situation. For example, one may feel angry at someone one longs for. The point is that from within any emotional perspective, certain aspects of reality are thematized and others escape one's attention.

to attribute to them a motivational basis in hope, curiosity, compassion, ambition, or another affect.

Because emotions are rooted in past experiences, they play an essential role in providing relevance to our activities; this same rootedness, however, can at times interfere with the important goal of reliably caring for all patients. For example, every physician has inadvertently spent too little time with some patients, compared with others with similar medical problems, because of feeling uncomfortable. And physicians preconsciously[4] modulate the amount of warmth or avoidance, both verbal and nonverbal, that they show patients according to their own past experiences with people the patient reminds them of. For example, the physician who learned to feel loving when holding the hand of an elderly grandparent may find herself taking her elderly patient's hand, moved by a loving feeling without any forethought. Similarly, the physician who learned to feel impotent rage toward an alcoholic father may find himself angrily avoiding the intoxicated person in the emergency room. Because experiences like this are ubiquitous, physicians need ways of managing their emotions to provide reliable care for all types of people.

Empathy Involves Using Resonance Emotions in the Service of Curiosity

It is because emotions carry one to familiar scenarios that they play an important role in empathy. In empathy, the thinkers' emotions *direct their attention*. What is unique about empathy is that the empathizers' current emotions are attuned to the emotions of another person through preverbal resonance, so that their attention can be directed to what is salient for the other person.

But there are important limits to how much resonance emotions contribute to empathy. First, the immediate shift in focus that occurs with resonance serves only as a clue (and not always an accurate one) to the general aspects of the patient's situation. By listening carefully to the patient's story and asking questions, one can capitalize on the suggestion. It is here, in the inquiry into what in particular is shaming *for the patient*, that the physician actually learns something new.

This is why Lipps's definition of empathy is potentially misleading for clinicians: for clinicians to project *themselves* into the patient's situation would distract them from learning how this other person actually feels. If resonance

---

4. I use the term *preconscious* here only to refer to subliminal experience. I refrain in this paper from discussing the large and interesting topic of whether there can be genuinely unconscious emotions.

feeling is not accompanied by a shift in focus to the patient's situation, empathic understanding is aborted. For example, an overwhelmingly fearful reaction of one's own can shift one's focus away from the details of the patient's situation. This sometimes happens when the patient's experience is too close to the physicians and invokes immediate personal concerns. For example, a physician who focuses on her own fear of breast cancer is likely to miss the particular meaning a mastectomy has for the patient.

Empathy necessarily involves dual perspectives, because one is both imaginatively in another's situation and also aware that this experience is not one's own but that of *another* person. This reflective aspect of empathy is one reason some see empathy as requiring emotional detachment. In contrast, I see this shift into a reflective stance as directed by the emotion of curiosity. In the case of Mr. L, I became curious about the resonance shame I felt in seeing his affliction. Rather than unreflectively acting on this shame and avoiding intruding on him, I was moved by curiosity to search for a more detailed understanding of why *he* might feel this way.

Aristotle and Plato's model of the curious person is the stargazer Thales, whose attention is directed toward the heavens rather than at his own footing on earth (Sokolowski 1988).[5] This model shows several aspects of curiosity. First, curious people are free of self-absorption—they lose themselves in whatever they contemplate. This does not imply that one ignores one's own personal reactions, as if they had no impact. Rather, one attempts to use one's own responses towards the goal of filling in the story the patient is telling, putting aside one's other issues when possible.

Second, Thales was not a specialist, and he was not passionately fixed on a particular object. Rather, his gaze was free to wander from star to star. This flexibility is essential if one is to follow a narrative imaginatively. Freud's image of the listening stance needed for analytic work is the passenger on a train gazing freely at the moving landscape.[6]

However, there are important limits to the usefulness of curiosity in empathic listening. Thales, Plato points out, is so absorbed in the stars that he falls into a well. If physicians' questions are not directed by resonance emotions, they

5. My discussion of curiosity and the use of Aristotle's model of the stargazer is particularly influenced by discussion with Karsten Harries, whose essay on "Truth and Freedom" includes some of this material.

6. Freud uses this image to describe free association to the analysand, but it applies equally well to the analyst, who Freud says is to have "evenly hovering attention" (Freud 1958, 12:111).

are likely to lose their grounding concerning what is significant for the patient. This in turn will make the patient feel like "a curiosity," rather than like someone who is being understood in a meaningful way. For example, if my curiosity about Mr. L was not guided by resonance with his feelings of helplessness and shame, I might have questioned him much more extensively in my first meetings with him, rather than enhancing his sense of control by asking him when I should return and how long he wanted to talk. Curiosity based in resonance emotion is more likely to respect the patient's needs. Resonance emotions are, after all, reminders that the physician actually shares the patient's human situation, including the shared possibilities of illness, suffering, and death. The empathic physician is thus more rooted than Thales, and less likely to fall into a well.

The idea that curiosity frees the physician's attention helps explain how physicians who are especially empathic may also be especially reliable and objective. When physicians feel *personally* threatened, enticed, or demoralized by their interactions with patients, their emotions threaten their role. In such cases, becoming curious about the patients decenters the physicians from their own emotional reactions without attenuating their interest in the patient. So, for example, the physician who feels angry at a patient who comes to the emergency room in the middle of the night for a "minor" complaint is more likely to get a good history, make an objective diagnosis, and treat the patient reliably if she becomes curious about why the patient feels her situation requires emergency care.

In addition, curiosity is much more useful than detachment for maintaining objectivity and reliability because physicians need to ensure not only that they do not overreact to patients, but also that they are not so distant that they fail to respond empathically. They are likely to lose information and efficacy by their inattentiveness and unsupportiveness in such cases. By becoming curious about their patterns of responding emotionally to patients, physicians can begin to correct for their own biases. When physicians notice their failures to resonate with certain types of patients, they can teach themselves to listen with curiosity to these patients' stories. And listening with curiosity to the story of a suffering person is likely to lead to the emotional resonance that is essential for empathy.

An additional benefit of becoming curious about one's own difficult emotional responses to patients is that such curiosity in and of itself often lightens the physician's burden. Rather than feeling that the situation with the patient just *is* scary, enraging, or seductive, the physician focuses on why these responses are happening now. This inquiry automatically reminds the physician that even intense emotions pass and can be managed in a variety of ways, thus freeing her to opt for a different approach to the patient. Although such inquiry (which I think is akin to empathizing with oneself) takes time to learn, it is not impossible to do within the current time constraints of medical practice.

Summary

Curiosity and resonance emotions meet in empathy, supplementing and correcting for each other's limitations. This helps account for some of the features of clinical empathy that have been difficult to explain. First, empathy involves using emotions for cognitive purposes. The notion that *experiencing* emotion is necessary to accurately *understand* someone challenges the ideal of "detached concern." This ideal presupposes that cognition and affect are entirely distinct faculties, but they are not. Resonance emotions play an essential role in directing the imaginative work of the empathizer.

Second, empathy and sympathy are related but distinct. They share a common precursor—both originate in resonance feeling. But in empathy, resonance emotions are used to understand another person more accurately, rather than to identify with her or take on her struggles as one's own.

Third, empathy happens spontaneously, and yet can be practiced and greatly enhanced over time. Empathy can be practiced "deliberately" despite the apparent spontaneity of resonance feelings, because one can develop the habit of responding to patients with curiosity about their lives.

Finally, even though emotions can bias and burden physicians, physicians who cultivate their capacities for curiosity and resonance are likely to be more reliable and objective. This is because empathy helps physicians understand patients and communicate better with them, which enhances diagnosis and treatment, and also because physicians can use their curiosity to disentangle themselves from some of the emotional reactions that threaten their role. For these reasons, physicians need to develop the emotional skills involved in empathy to practice more effective, and not just more pleasing, medicine.

References

Aring, C. 1958. Sympathy and empathy. *Journal of the American Medical Association.* 167:448–52.

Beauchamp, T., and J. Childress. 1979. *Principles of Biomedical Ethics.* New York: Oxford University Press.

Blumgart, H. 1964. Caring for the patient. *New England Journal of Medicine.* 270:449–56.

deSousa, R. 1987. *The Rationality of Emotion.* Cambridge: MIT Press.

Fox, R., and H. Lief. 1963. Training for "detached concern." In *The Psychological Basis of Medical Practice,* ed. H. Lief and Lief. New York: Harper and Row.

Freud, S. 1953–74. *The Standard Edition of the Complete Psychological Works of Sigmund Freud*. Ed. and trans. J. Strachey. 23 vols. London: Hogarth Press.

Hunsdahl, J. 1967. Concerning Einfühlung (empathy): A concept of its origin and early development. *Journal of the History of the Behavioral Sciences*. 3:180–91.

Sawyier, R. 1974. A conceptual analysis of empathy. *Annual of Psychoanalysis*. 3:37–47.

Sokolowski, R., ed. 1988. *Edmund Husserl and the Phenomenological Tradition: Essays in Phenomenology*. Washington, D.C.: Catholic University of America Press.

Spiro, H. 1986. *Doctors, Patients and Placebos*. New Haven: Yale University Press.

Chapter 16
Empathic Immersion

PETER KRAMER

Modern forms of psychotherapy use empathy as their sole foundation, but empathy is an elusive concept to build on. How much weight can empathy bear?

I think, for example, of a Boston psychoanalyst whose patient, an angry young woman, ranted at her throughout many months of treatment (Stark in press). A keen sense of attunement led the analyst to understand that the woman perceived her as a depriving parent. Time and time again, the analyst calmly and kindly pointed out this confusion. The therapy progressed, but only slowly. Finally the patient "got to" the analyst. In response to a goading comment, the analyst exploded with rage of her own. The patient experienced immense relief. The pace of the therapy quickened. The patient felt appreciated at last. Which was empathy—the attuned understanding or the rage?

We associate empathy with sweetness—"soothing" is the word generally used to described empathy's effect—but empathy disconcerts as often as it comforts. Some years ago, I attended a seminar on hypnosis. In the initial exercise, I was coupled with a psychologist I had never met before. She was well-dressed and had a mature and confident look about her. We were instructed to

I wish to thank Drs. Diana Lidofsky and Paul Ornstein, who were kind enough to discuss some of the clinical material in this chapter with me.

engage in a relaxation technique, one that entailed my monitoring my partner's feelings as she focused first on the sounds around her and then on her bodily state. As the exercise progressed, I developed a disturbing impression of this woman. Though her words were about sensory perceptions of external stimuli, I became aware that she was suffering inwardly from a terrible feeling of vulnerability. I experienced her unease as a visceral sensation in my chest. There arose in me as well certain cruel impulses; I felt empowered, believing I could injure her. I surmised social masochism must be ruining her life. At the end of the induction, each member of the pair was to say what he or she had learned about the other. We were both too shaken to proceed. At last I said, "I hope you are in therapy for this problem," and she nodded that she was.

For me, that moment typifies the empathic interaction: it is often surprising. At this moment, we see the other person anew. But empathy is not limited to the observer's cognition. Empathy is action as well—to be understood is unsettling. Nor is empathy simple in its form. It is not merely imitative, reproducing in one what the other feels. Empathy also consists of complementary states, like sadism in response to masochism. And empathy can be learned or enhanced, even through quite mechanical exercises, so that it can occur without any intention to lend support.

This being said, I should add that for certain people, and I count myself among them, there is an appealing, even an addictive, quality about intimate attunement to another person. The allure of "sailing close to the wind" (Kramer 1989, 246) or singing "close to the music of what happens" (Heaney quoted in Havens 1989, 153) has always drawn to the profession of psychiatry people whose temperament and early experience—some say rearing by a depressed mother is a crucial factor (Storr 1979, 174)—lead them to be adept at amplifying small interpersonal cues.

But although empathy is one of psychiatry's rewards, for years it was a secret pleasure, incidental to the more general task of making sense of the patient's character and illness. For much of modern psychotherapy's first century, empathy played only a limited role.

Sigmund Freud, although he maintained a friendly relationship with many of his analysands (Wolf 1991, 185–97; Kohut 1977, 255–56), recommended that analysts conduct treatment in the emotional equivalent of a sterile field: "I cannot advise my colleagues too urgently to model themselves during psychoanalytic treatment on the surgeon, who puts aside all his feelings, even his human sympathy, and concentrates his mental forces on the single aim of performing the operations as skillfully as possible. . . . The justification for requiring this emotional coldness in the analyst is that it creates the most advantageous conditions for both parties" (Freud 1912, 115).

Freud rarely referred to "empathy" (*Einfühlung*), a word that at the turn of the century was still reserved primarily for the feelings with which an observer invested a work of art (Jackson 1992). Freud did use the term in a discussion of group psychotherapy, where he noted the utility, perhaps the indispensability, of empathy for comprehending another's emotional life (Freud 1921, 108; Basch 1983, 103). But there were other ways to approach patients, through the whole complex paraphernalia of psychoanalysis, from dream interpretation to the associative reconstruction of childhood trauma. Though psychoanalysis "transformed the intuitive empathy of artists and poets into the observational tool of a trained scientific investigator" (Kohut 1971, 303), empathy represented but one of many routes to cognitive understanding of the other's circumstances.

Over the years, empathy has assumed an increasingly important place in classical psychoanalysis, particularly through emphasis on the need for analysts to be aware of the emotional screen through which they see patients. But the goal of classical psychoanalysis remains transformation through insight—resolving unacknowledged inner conflict, making the unconscious conscious, and giving the rational mind dominance over the irrational. In this schema, empathy does not cure; it serves as a source of information (one of many, and a sometimes suspect one at that) (Basch 1983, 101) for the doctor about the patient.

Empathy-as-action is another matter. It is only in recent years that psychotherapists have begun to rely on empathy's power to do something—to influence the patient's feelings, especially the patient's feelings about the self (self-esteem, self-confidence, and so on). The most important new offshoot of psychoanalysis, "self-psychology," deemphasizes the importance of patients' growth in understanding and instead stresses the curative power of the patient's feeling understood, by an empathic therapist.

The pioneering figure in self-psychology is the late Heinz Kohut, a Viennese-born, Chicago-based analyst who found himself frustrated by his patients' incomplete response to Freudian treatments. Kohut came to believe that what ailed his patients was not so much conflict—id versus ego, wish versus fear—as deficits in the self. Kohut was especially interested in self-centered, needy, narcissistic people who formed an increasing proportion of patients in his analytic practice. When his patients—who often suffered from chronic mood disturbances and were quite difficult to treat—said they felt empty or that something was missing within them, Kohut began to take these statements quite literally.

The problem was not that conflict caused these patients to repress feelings, but rather that something had gone wrong in the course of their development. The issue was not guilt or anxiety but deprivation (Lee and Martin 1991, 191–

93). Much of the modern popular impression of what is wrong with people when they feel lost and inadequate—apparent in the teachings of Adult Children of Alcoholics and other movements that emphasize the destructive power of parental neglect—finds its implicit intellectual underpinnings in Kohut's writings.

Kohut began, like a classical psychoanalyst, to use empathy as a source of information, but he took this principle to its limits. Kohut diagnosed patients entirely according to the empathic hinder they showed in treatment—whether they seemed to long for a mother's love, a father's direction, or a sibling's playfulness. Most often, the deficit was in parental (traditionally maternal) responsiveness. Typically, the narcissistic patient would have been raised by an equally injured narcissistic mother who could not transcend her own needs and therefore could not see her child accurately.

The central image in self-psychology—the image of what makes development go right—is the "gleam in the mother's eyes, which mirrors the child's exhibitionistic display (Kohut 1971, 116). In the growing child, a healthy sense of self arises from parental attunement. Self-psychological psychotherapy responds to the deficits created by unattuned parenting. This is Kohut's second, and revolutionary, use of empathy. He began to turn to empathy—what I have called empathy-as-action—as the central source of cure in treatment. The self-psychological therapist accepts and indulges the patient's need to be seen accurately and benignly, even to be admired—a process called "mirroring."

The Kohutian analyst's plan is not to resolve conflict (even the Oedipus conflict, the story at the heart of classical psychoanalysis, becomes secondary [Kohut 1977, 220–48]); rather, the analyst struggles to attain empathic attunement, often with quite difficult-to-like patients, believing that "mirroring" right in the therapy—responding with consistent, appropriate admiration—will allow the patient to resume previously stunted growth. Conflicts then resolve spontaneously. In the restored self, dynamic tensions dissipate.

Kohut saw all people as existing in a social world. Throughout life, a person will use aspects of others as part of the inner self. A favored example is the child who can ice-skate better if the parent skates nearby; psychologically, the parent provides confidence or balance, functions normally understood as intrapsychic (Tolpin 1983, 363–79). The self-psychological analyst does not worry much about the patient's dependency. It is appropriate for analysis to have a "firming" function—think, again, of firming of the ankles—and for the patient to learn what it is like to need and trust another person. Just as "You never outgrow your need for milk," people never outgrow their need for others to foster certain internal functions (Baker and Baker 1987). For Kohut, the goal of treatment was not independence but mature interdependence, nourished by "empathic intuneness" between the self and sustaining aspects of others (Kohut 1984, 65–66). Thus, beyond its roles as diagnostic and therapeutic tool, empathy has additional roles in self-psychology, as a sustainer and marker of health in relations between aspects of the self and between self and others.

Although the moment-to-moment practice of self-psychology may look like Freudian psychoanalysis, the break with tradition is quite radical. Self-psychology is not a "psychodynamic psychotherapy" because what is dynamic in the patient—anxiety, resulting from conflicting impulses—is deemed unimportant. And self-psychology ignores or denies the role of certain of the patient's own drives in causing illness; in particular, self-psychology has little use for the concept of innate aggression. The self-psychologist sees the patient as injured through deprivation, not as hostile or sexually driven. Implicit is a positive, optimistic view of human nature. The untraumatized individual is naturally empathic.

In brief, self-psychology forgoes the entire apparatus of traditional psychotherapy's structure of mind (ego, id, superego), drives (sexuality, aggression), pathology (repressed conflict), method of cure (insight by making the unconscious conscious), and goal of treatment (mature independence). Instead, for self-psychology, failures and treatment of mental disorder, and the capacity for empathy, serves as the key marker and sustainer of mental health.

Certain of Kohut's followers today, the "intersubjective" school, place even more emphasis on empathy than Kohut did (Storolow et al. 1987). They believe that the *only* proper stance of the analyst is what Kohut called "protracted empathic immersion" (Kohut 1977, 302).

While Kohut discarded many of Freud's assumptions and practices, he still believed that therapists should keep their patients feeling somewhat frustrated in their needs. That is, Kohut continued to accept the principle of "optimal frustration"—although what Kohut considered optimal entailed a good deal more open warmth than was provided by typical classical psychoanalysts of mid-century. Much of the contemporary emphasis on the good therapist's "availability" and responsiveness is traceable to Kohut's ideas.

Kohut's more radical followers, the intersubjective psychoanalysts, have discarded the goal of optimal frustration and aim instead for maximal empathic resonance—optimal attunement or optimal responsiveness—on the part of the therapist. Unlike Freud and Kohut, the intersubjective self-psychologist does not oscillate between empathic and objective or external modes of viewing the patient. Intersubjective self-psychology holds that "psychoanalytic investigation is *always* from within a subjective world," that is, in the absence of any objective knowledge of the patient's life (Storolow et al. 1987, 5–6). Not only does empathy play the central role in pathology, diagnosis, and recovery, the good therapist's stance—or vision—is purely and consistently one of empathy.

In an era that increasingly values empathy, it is instructive to consider the consequences of a treatment that relies on empathy and demands that the therapist forgo many other possible responses. For instance, the therapist must ignore awareness of social norms. When the patient does something patently unreasonable, the therapist should not want to say, "But can't you see how that appears to others!" Instead, the therapist will resonate with the fear of decompensation that gave rise to the strikingly self-centered behavior.

For instance: a patient has a particularly rewarding session with his analyst.[1] At the next meeting, the analyst enters the waiting room from a different door than he uses ordinarily, and the patient spends the hour ranting about the analyst's terrible unreliability—does the analyst not know that constancy is the basis of all treatment? Ignoring the external viewpoint, the analyst moves to understand the patient's response from within—from the "empathic vantage"—agreeing that inconstancy is enraging. Feeling understood and accepted, the patient responds with a fresh nugget of self-awareness. When the analyst came in by the wrong door, the patient realized the analyst has a private life and probably had not, as the patient wished, spent the whole night thinking about the prior rewarding session. Thus, entering by the wrong door was an "empathic rupture," a dashing of the patient's hope of being held constantly in the parent's gaze.

It is quite wonderful to hear reports of self-psychologists under attack by aggressively obnoxious patients. The therapist avoids any recourse to reason (or even to the interpersonal context—"You make me feel threatened") and instead helps elaborate the patient's expression of frustration (Kramer 1990, 4–5). Sustained empathy—rather like the sustained holding that has been recommended for autistic and even normal children (Welch 1988)—can have a transformative effect for patients. Being understood is an enveloping sensation that facilitates access to painful, forgotten, or even unformed, prohibited feelings; this process, along with the patient's ongoing use of the therapist for various inner functions (such as confidence, resilience, or even self-worth) promotes growth.

Self-psychology's highlighting of empathy has resulted in many powerful episodes of psychotherapy. But problems arise when we try to understand in a systematic way just what constitutes empathic treatment.

Consider the following contretemps: a young woman consults a female psychiatrist for problems of low self-worth and intercurrent depression. As a child, the patient was shunted from one psychotherapist to another by a superficially supportive mother whom the girl experienced as uncaring and judgmental. Each therapy referral made the girl feel naughty and defective. The child turned away from the mother toward a distant, demanding father. Today, she under-

1. Paul Ornstein provided me with this example.

stands her obsessive efforts in graduate school motivated by an immature need to please him.

On a trip home, the young woman presents her academic progress to her father, and he scorns it as meager and inadequate. In the following session, the patient describes this encounter. Believing she feels some of the young woman's distress, the psychiatrist exclaims, "How painful for you!" Far from showing signs of being comforted, the patient attacks the psychiatrist, "I would never have thought this of you! You're just like my mother—always thinking I'm helpless." Furious at the psychiatrist's insensitivity, the patient seethes for the rest of the session.

Such misunderstandings are common. What do we make of them? I discussed this moment in therapy with two self-psychologists—the treating clinician and a senior consultant. The treating therapist was under the impression that she had cut too close to the bone. The patient was, indeed, in terrible pain, and the bald naming of the emotion shamed the patient and threw her into rageful denial.

This reading of the situation creates a problem for self-psychology. The therapist spoke from a empathic vantage, but the result was further pain and alienation for the patient. Kohut was aware of this problem, and in his last book he wrote that in analysis, as in life, "the desideratum is exposure to attenuated empathy, not exposure to total and all-encompassing empathy," which can overwhelm or "flood" the patient, as perhaps the patient was flooded by a parent's panic in the face of minor sadness or anxiety the patient displayed in childhood (Kohut 1984, 82).

The senior consultant saw the vignette differently. He believed that the interpretation addressed the patient at the wrong level. The patient was perhaps not aware that the father had caused her pain. If the therapist had said something more tentative—"Your father's response disturbed you?"—she might have learned that nearer to the level of awareness the patient had a different response to the father's behavior than the therapist anticipated. The patient might have said she appreciated her father's accurate assessment of her shortcomings. The consultant's critique introduces a new complexity, the idea of levels of empathy. It also admits a degree of circularity. That comment is empathic which is experienced and acknowledged by the patient as empathic.

This definition of "being empathic" is in fact one self-psychology has adopted. "Being empathic is an interpersonal response occurring between the therapist and the patient by which the therapist uses his or her empathy to voice comments about this patient's internal state, which results in the patient's feeling understood and soothed" (Book 1988, 421). (Another approach is to equate empathy with "perfect courtesy" or "tact" [Kohut 1977, 258–59]). In other words, we know an action is empathic because it is comforting to the patient.

Not all actions that arise from empathy qualify as "empathic." A therapist might come to understand, by means of empathy, that a patient is dangerous and should be committed involuntarily. If the resultant action were experienced by the patient as soothing, it would be empathic; if not, not (Book 1989). Indeed, even attunement to the patient will not be empathic—nor should we expect it to be therapeutic—if it is not simultaneously soothing. Soothing is the test, the criterion, of empathy-as-action.

While this approach settles the case of the graduate student—since the interpretation induced seething, instead of soothing, it was not empathic—it raises a host of questions. Must patients always be soothed? Must therapists never insist on an interpretation with which a patient initially disagrees? Has confrontation no role in psychotherapy? And how shall we value all those early therapies that aimed to unsettle, rather than to comfort?

Here is a difficult situation. Self-psychology bases all aspects of healing on empathy. Since empathy has so many aspects—can often be disturbing or even destructive—self-psychologists have introduced the criterion of soothing. But this new parameter impoverishes empathy, acknowledges empathy only of the palest, most Pollyannaish sort.

As critics have argued, there is a "dark side of empathy" (Modell 1986) that self-psychology denies or fails to use. I have presented elsewhere (Kramer 1989, 142) a vignette in which an empathic encounter centered on sexual disgust. In listening to a woman who consulted me about low self-esteem, I found my mind wandering to a white excrescence I had just found on the leaves of an office plant infested with mealybug. Asking myself why, I was struck with the notion that I was experiencing a version of the sexual self-loathing that was inhibiting my patient. I raised this issue, and the therapy moved ahead. While this process was liberating in the long run—progress depended on the patient's bringing into consciousness and reconsidering her self-disgust—when I first expressed my awareness of what troubled her, the patient felt deep discomfort, even shame.

Empathy is often undue intimacy—knowing something the other is not aware of having revealed, perhaps even something the other is unaware of having thought or felt. As such, it can be disturbing, to both parties. The closeness that intimate awareness brings can make us squirm, which is why the attenuation of empathy in ordinary life (and in much of medicine outside psychotherapy) is so marked. With regard to empathy as a perceptual route, we often wear blinders or earplugs, for fear that we sense too much. If empathy must always soothe, then self-psychologists, the most empathic of therapists, may function best if within psychotherapy they engage in self-handicapping of this sort.

That it soothe is a restricted, not to say peculiar, criterion for empathy. The existential psychotherapist Leston Havens lists a series of tests of empathy

(Havens 1986, 18–20). In motor empathy, one finds oneself assuming the posture of the other. (Family therapists use this technique quite purposefully, for instance, altering power relations in the family by mimicking the weak and passive father, who then becomes endowed with some of the therapist's status.) In affective empathy, one reflects inwardly the mood expressed by the other's demeanor. Cognitive empathy is tested by attempting silently to anticipate or complete the patient's sentences, and the test is that one does so successfully. In perceptual empathy—perhaps the most complete and noble form—the therapist sees the patient afresh, often experiencing astonishment in the process.

These tests are largely internal to the therapist. They allow for what we might call value-free empathy, a knowing of the other that does not favor comforting over challenging, reassuring over embarrassing. The success of reaching the patient through empathy is ultimately verified by the patient's response, but that response may be of a variety of sorts. Traditionally, psychotherapists have believed an intervention is on target if it elicits new material from the patient; the test of accuracy is not soothing but stimulating. Just as the therapist's empathy may shock, startle, or instruct the patient, the patient's response to effective empathy will often surprise the therapist and redirect the treatment.

The exclusive focus on empathy diminishes both participants, demanding that therapists ignore many of their own human strengths and, in parallel fashion, ignore sources of resilience in their patients. It is intriguing to contrast intersubjective self-psychology with another important strain of psychoanalysis, one that also begins with the assumption that psychotherapy takes place in the equal interplay between therapist and patient. I have in mind interpersonal psychoanalysis, the heritage of the innovative American psychoanalyst Harry Stack Sullivan.

Interpersonal psychoanalysis attends to social behavior, and the analyst will often point out how the patient's attitude or behavior strikes other people. In particular, the analyst is free to let the patient know how one or another action affects him or her (the analyst). The analyst is thus simultaneously aware of how the patient feels and how it feels to be with the patient. The interpersonal psychoanalyst Philip Bromberg complains that in focusing "only on what the patient needs from the analyst, or, how it feels to be the subject *rather* than the target of the patient's needs and demands . . . a self psychologist [functions] as if he were an interpersonal analyst who is deaf in one ear (Bromberg 1989, 286). The self-psychologist assumes that any failures in the empathic encounter arise from the analyst's own insensitivity, as if the patient's resistance did not matter at all. In requiring nothing of the patient and everything of the therapist, self-psychology implies that the analyst is a more complete person than the patient (ibid.). And even if the analyst succeeds in conveying perfect empathy, this success may inhibit the creativity of the patient who has, in effect, been made passive by self-psychology's assumptions about the unidirectional nature of empathic effort (Modell 1986).

In interpersonal psychoanalysis, the analyst sometimes takes a quite anti-empathic stance. In order to discourage the patient from repeating the maladaptive social behavior, the analyst may intentionally frustrate the patient's expectations, perhaps responding in a distant fashion just when the patient expects to be met with warmth. This strategy is called counterprojective technique—blocking the feelings and behaviors that the patient ordinarily projects onto authority figures. Deprived of the usual scenario, the patient is thrown back on his or her own resources and is forced to own rather than project anger and anxiety.

More broadly, the demand for constant soothing empathy limits the parts of the therapist's self that come into play. The traditional psychoanalyst is not so much supportive as inquisitive—a sort of co-explorer on a journey in which quite terrible things may be learned, not the least of which concern the explorers themselves. To be sure, this undertaking requires that the patient trust the therapist: classical analysts refer to the "therapeutic alliance," in which the analyst displays enough reliable human qualities for the enterprise to proceed.

Still, the traditional therapeutic attitude is well characterized in John Updike's likening of the editor William Shawn to a Freudian psychoanalyst: "an infinitely patient expectancy was the mood he conveyed, and it was this expectancy, grandly nondirective, that a contributor longed to satisfy. [Shawn established] an air of perfect listening, in which you were encouraged to reveal and reconstruct yourself" (Updike 1992–93, 141). The traditional analyst may show more of the father's raised eyebrow than the mother's twinkling eye. Empathy is used to recognize deception and self-deception, to challenge as much as to soothe. Indeed, if the process of self-exploration becomes too consistently soothing, then the process itself must be examined and interpreted. My own psychoanalysis, the one in which I was a patient, was of this sort; my gratitude for that therapy is no doubt one element in my reluctance to embrace empathy as the "royal road" to transformation.

The curative stance can be less soothing yet. Franz Alexander, the psychoanalytic pioneer in psychosomatics, was said to have been unperturbed if patients hated him. Being able to hate the analyst is a sign of independence; it follows that the patient need not be overly afraid of angering the analyst, nor should the analyst flinch from being hated, so long as the patient undergoes growth. Even the analyst's own aggressive impulses have their uses: to the child psychoanalyst D. W. Winnicott, by all accounts the most empathic of therapists, is attributed the aphorism that any patient who has not been hated by his analyst has been cheated.

One of the most beautiful stories I know about the complex relationship of empathy to psychotherapy is told by the poet and animal trainer Vicki Hearne concerning a thoroughbred named Drummer Girl (Hearne 1986, 117–54). In her early years, Drummer Girl was inconsistently trained and ridden—Hearne gives the impression that Drummer Girl suffered in the way that sensitive children do in response to rearing by narcissistic parents. As a result, Drummer Girl mistrusted the usual tender gestures with which people woo horses: "She had especially had it with kindness, any story about kindness. One of the many things that inspired terror and rage was a soothing pat on the shoulder" (ibid., 128).

When it came to jumps, Drummer Girl was a fence rusher. Hearne trained her by letting her rush fences, but then, just after the jump, bringing her up short with a "halt correction." Because Drummer Girl, for all her touchiness, had what Hearne calls a moral sensibility—a sense of grace and balance—the horse began to anticipate the halt after the jump. She dropped her fence rushing and in time began to canter into an approach that resulted in a supple jump that gave her control on the far side of the barrier. The further consequence was that in many areas of her life, this once unruly, seemingly vicious horse came to choose a "muscular version of the good" over her former chaotic behavior (ibid., 138–39).

How shall we class Hearne's intervention? It is based on a combination of empathic knowledge and identification (Hearne says that without the satisfaction that animal training gives her, she might be as self-destructive as her "crazy horses" [ibid., 139–40]). Most obviously, it arises from expert knowledge, both the teacher's ability to identify a promising troubled pupil and her knack for packaging a lesson in the student's own metaphor, in this case the primacy of body grace. There is also an element of active joining: Hearne believes Drummer Girl at first sees her interventions to be the acts of a crazy woman, which is to say a kindred spirit.

Hearne's saving of Drummer Girl from fear and rage embodies what Havens has called "active empathy"—Havens uses Martin Buber's phrase, "a 'bold swinging . . . into the life of the other'"—so different from the passive empathy of the waiting, sentient, echoing listener (Havens 1986, 16–17). Here, empathy is something like speaking the patient's language (Kramer 1989, 129–53), even if the initial result is far from soothing. If the basis for therapy is "making contact" or "engaging the patient," then empathic immersion—in the sense of remaining strictly within the patient's perspective—is but one way to meet that requirement.

I mention Drummer Girl because I believe her treatment has parallels with a well-known case from the self-psychology literature (Storolow et al. 1987, 144–55; Kramer 1993). The case involves a psychotic young woman who in childhood suffered so many terrible losses—including her father's suicide—that she began to feel Christ had abandoned her. By her later twenties, she considered herself to be a member of the Holy Trinity through whom God's love is transmitted to a cruel world. After consulting a counselor who proved exploitative, she turned to an "intersubjective" psychoanalyst, one who believed, as many self-psychologists do today, that the principle of empathic immersion should be applied to a broad range of patients, not just those who might be diagnosed as "narcissistic."

The analyst tried to focus on this patient's human qualities. But the analyst was not speaking her language, not engaging her over her religious preoccupation, so he failed. The patient announced a plan to enter into a state of meditation and prayer that would hasten the Second Coming. The therapist expressed reservations, and this protective gesture was again experienced as a failure of empathy. The patient demanded that the analyst pick up the phone and arrange for her to meet again with the exploitative counselor, whom she saw as Christ.

As this point, the analyst, understanding that his approach had misfired, reversed course. He interrupted the patient's religious ruminations and demanded her attention. He said there would be no meeting with the exploitative counselor. Instead, the analyst announced that he had his own plan, "a plan in which she would become well again and return to live with the people who loved her . . . [and] that he was himself the only person in this world she should be concerned about seeing, for it was in their work together that the goal of this new plan would be attained" (Storolow et al. 1987, 153). The patient cried for twenty minutes and then ended the appointment. But soon her religious preoccupations diminished.

In other words, the analyst abruptly halted the patient's characteristic behavior. He entered into her world and contracted to become her savior, perhaps even her Savior.

I have mentioned a parallel between Drummer Girl's treatment and that of this patient. The parallel I see is that for both patients "empathy," in the commonest sense—reassurance and sympathy—was poison. Both required a dramatic "correction," an attention-catching intervention that indicated that the therapist was different, even crazy in a certain way. And both responded to this craziness with complementary grace, a demonstration of unknown, perhaps repressed, capacities.

The case of this psychotic young woman gives us a window on the practical world of therapeutic empathy. It confirms the observation that the stance we would ordinarily call empathic is rarely enough. In this case, gentle attunement to the persisting human qualities proved a failed strategy. The patient's response also calls into question the centrality of soothing. To be sure, the patient ultimately comes to feel safe—as patients also do in therapies in which empathy is a peripheral consideration—but she is overwhelmed at first. Indeed, we may wonder whether her response to the therapist's new firmness and vigor is not astonishment. Soothing "in due time" is a new standard; soothing becomes less a measure of the immediate intervention than a goal—perhaps one among many—of the therapy as a whole.

This case also reopens the question that has stuck with us all along: what does it mean to be empathic? Accepting baptism, the analyst rejects or ignores many empathic alternatives. For instance, he chooses to block the patient's attachment to the exploitative counselor, when it might be argued that the empathic stance would be to side understandingly with her masochism. The analyst declines to adopt the patient's eschatological expectations; perhaps a more strictly empathic posture would involve joining her in the belief that the world is about to end. Judging the treatment by the standard of the absolute empathic vantage, we may wonder whether the analyst has not cheated a bit, by taking into account private beliefs—the world spins on, the counselor is dangerous—that are quite distinct from and external to what the patient feels.

We might even say that the analyst's stance with regard to the patient, like the trainer's with regard to Drummer Girl, is counterprojective (in the tradition of Harry Stack Sullivan). To both patients, the traditionally "empathic" role represents a threat of abandonment or exploitation. The intersubjective analyst's dramatic change in role blocks the patient's projection: "You appear kind, therefore you will disappoint me." The analyst forcefully declares himself to be distinct from the patient's past love objects. This extreme form of empathy—choosing to embody certain of a patient's deepest wishes—may not even be experienced as empathy. Like matter at extreme velocity or with extreme mass, empathy under extreme conditions may take on strange properties.

For example, to be faced with a doctor who promises to save her may be disarming. That is, it may rob the patient of her characteristic defenses (to choose men poorly, long for Christ, and reenact past injuries). Bypassing the defenses is a complex act. Consider the feelings of an angry patient whose rage a counterproductive therapist mimics or adopts—agreeing with the patient's outrage. To have someone don your very own character armor can leave you denuded, alone with the self. The patient is stripped of any ordinary form of self-support, namely distance from people who deny the validity of any angry feelings. In the extreme, empathy with rage is a form of confrontation—it precipitates a confrontation of the self by the self. The analyst's assuming an ideal role in the patient's psychotic fantasy may have a quite similar effect. The intervention remains clever and perhaps even empathic (it may seem more grounded in intuition than empathy), but it may work through a variety of means—function as confrontation or insight, or some other, less easily specified, form of self-awareness.

My own sense is that empathy properly takes on many roles in psychotherapy. In the therapeutic encounter both therapist and patient put the tools at hand to many uses. Patients quite commonly incorporate interpretation as support, experiencing not the specifics of what the therapist says but rather a general sensation of being cared for and attended to (Kramer 1989, 81–105); equally, a patient may understand support as insight, thinking, "If my therapist supports me, I must be worthy," or "I must be needy."

The more we look as the decision to save the psychotic young woman on her terms, the stranger it seems. It has the quality of shaking her by the shoulders and saying, "Don't you see I love you." Along with the promise of dedication, it may even contain a touch of the sadism that this patient elicits from others. I suspect the intervention succeeds not because it soothes but because it reaches this patient at all. The key factor is making contact.

Engagement is a central function of empathy-as-action: patients are hard to reach, harder than we generally imagine. Empathy is a way both of locating patients and helping them feel the therapist's presence. There are, of course, other ways to contact patients; many of the "strategies" of strategic psychotherapy have this goal. In this sense, empathy-as-action is but one tool among many for fulfilling the precondition of psychotherapy, just as "vicarious introspection," as Kohut characterized empathy (Kohut 1959, 463), is but one tool for coming to understand patients. As for "being empathic," perhaps it is a term best dropped from the technical lexicon. Empathy is attunement, a state that arouses a variety of responses from the comfortable to the unbearable. Soothing is a poor test of empathy, and the question whether soothing is a preferred intervention in psychotherapy is an empirical one, separable from the issue of how far the therapist's actions ought to be informed by or built upon empathic awareness.

At the same time, it seems important to acknowledge the restorative effect of self-psychology on psychotherapy. The effort to build a psychotherapy on empathy is an inspired act of intellectual creativity. Outside self-psychology, it has influenced psychotherapists to reassess the importance of empathy, and in so doing to question the authority and wisdom of the analyst whose aim is to reconstruct childhood history or to help patients reconcile conflicting impulses. It has also contributed to the current awareness of the deprivation that results from neglect and abuse in childhood. Inside self-psychology, the emphasis on empathy has given rise to treatments of inspiring consistency and great beauty.

What goes on in those therapies—I mean what goes on from the viewpoint of the patient—remains an interesting question. That the therapist's vantage is empathic does not guarantee that the transformational element in the treatment is empathy. Our culture is one in which empathic encounters are almost always attenuated. The relentlessly empathic therapist may seem to the patient to be a person of unusual powers, an alien creature—perhaps one who through a refusal to fight or to flee pushes the patient into a difficult self-examination. In the end, empathy, for all its special virtues, is a form of contact between flawed humans, and it seems unlikely that in the interchange the usual issues of aggression, shame, and longing should be absent.

References

Baker, H. S., and M. N. Baker. 1987. Heinz Kohut's self psychology: An overview. *American Journal of Psychiatry.* 144:1–9.

Basch, M. F. 1983. Empathic understanding: A review of the concept and some theoretical considerations. *Journal of the American Psychoanalytic Association.* 31(1):101–26.

Book, H. E. 1988. Empathy: Misconceptions and misuses in psychotherapy. *American Journal of Psychiatry.* 145:420–24.

Book, H. E. 1989. The meaning of empathy. *American Journal of Psychiatry.* 146:413–14.

Bromberg, P. W. 1989. "Interpersonal psychoanalysis and self psychology: A clinical comparison." In *Self Psychology: Comparisons and Contrasts*, ed. D. W. Detrick and S. P. Detrick. Hillsdale, N.J.: Analytic Press.

Freud, S. 1912. Recommendations to physicians practicing psychoanalysis. In *The Standard Edition of the Complete Psychological Works of Sigmund Freud*, ed. and trans. J. Strachey, vol. 12. London: Hogarth Press.

Freud, S. 1921. Group psychology and the analysis of the ego. In *The Standard Edition of the Complete Psychological Works of Sigmund Freud*, ed. and trans. J. Strachey, vol. 17. London: Hogarth Press.

Havens, L. 1986. *Making Contact: Uses of Language in Psychotherapy.* Cambridge, Mass.: Harvard University Press.

Havens, L. 1989. *A Safe Place: Laying the Groundwork of Psychotherapy.* Cambridge, Mass.: Harvard University Press.

Hearne, V. 1986. *Adam's Task: Calling Animals by Name.* New York: Knopf.

Jackson, S. W. 1992. The listening healer in the history of psychological healing. *American Journal of Psychiatry.* 149:1623–32.

Kohut, H. 1959. Introspection, empathy, and psychoanalysis: An examination of the relationship between mode of observation and theory. *Journal of the American Psychoanalytic Association.* 7:459–83.

Kohut, H. 1971. *The Analysis of the Self: A Systematic Approach to the Psychoanalytic Treatment of Narcissistic Personality Disorders.* New York: International Universities Press.

Kohut, H. 1977. *The Restoration of the Self.* New York: International Universities Press.

Kohut, H. 1984. *How Does Analysis Cure?* Ed. A. Goldberg and P. E. Stepansky. Chicago: University of Chicago Press.

Kramer, P. D. 1989. *Moments of Engagement: Intimate Psychotherapy in a Technological Age.* New York: W. W. Norton.

Kramer, P. D. 1990. Cosi fan tutte. *Psychiatric Times.* April:4–5.

Kramer, P. D. 1993. Amazing grace. *Psychiatric Times.* In press.

Lee, R. R., and J. C. Martin. 1991. *Psychotherapy after Kohut: A Textbook of Self Psychology.* Hillsdale, N.J.: Analytic Press.

Modell, A. 1986. The missing elements in Kohut's cure. *Psychoanalytic Inquiry.* 6:367–85.

Stark, M. (In press). *Psychotherapeutic Technique: Working with the Resistance.* New York: Jason Aronson.

Storolow, R. D., B. Brandschaft, and G. Atwood. 1987. *Psychoanalytic Treatment: An Intersubjective Approach.* Hillsdale, N.J.: Analytic Press.

Storr, A. 1979. *The Art of Psychotherapy.* London: Secker and Warburg.

Tolpin, M. 1983. Corrective emotional experience: A self psychological reevaluation. In *The Future of Psychoanalysis: Essays in Honor of Heinz Kohut,* ed. A. Goldberg. New York: International Universities Press.

Updike, J. 1992–93. "Remembering Mr. Shawn." *New Yorker.* 28 December 1992/ 4 January 1993:141.

Welch, M. C. 1988. *Holding Time.* New York: Simon and Schuster.

Wolf, E. S. 1991. Heinz Kohut memorial lecture: Toward a level playing field. In *The Evolution of Self Psychology: Progress in Self Psychology,* ed. A. Goldberg. Hillsdale, N.J.: Analytic Press.

Chapter 17
Epilogue

The message of this book is simple: good clinicians use all kinds of information about their patients; they listen as well as look. However great the triumphs of science, some things remain unseen. Thanks to technology, the physician's gaze has turned from the patient as a person to the organs, cells, and molecules within; the body is in danger of disappearing along with mind and spirit. Medical students are selected for their grades and trained scientifically to use their eyes and not their ears; they are put to work in hospitals where knowing what pills to give and how to wield a scalpel saves more lives than the character of a physician.

Of course, until a few decades ago, physicians could only *care* for their patients; now the chance to *cure* so many makes science and technology irresistible, and essential. Patients know this and rightly demand a scientific approach to their problems. They want easy answers, too. No one wants to feel responsible for his or her travails. Where once someone with a peptic ulcer took that diagnosis as a warning against working too hard, having the wrong goals, or being under "stress," today the discovery of *H. pylori*, those alien bacteria in the interstices of the stomach, provide a new excuse. "It's not me, it's my mucus," absolves people of any need to change. Moreover, medications developed in the last twenty years have made it so easy to heal a peptic ulcer that the doctor looks

190

only at the ulcer crater and not at the patient. Ulcers are readily healed, but their origin in mind and spirit, as well as in mucus, is forgotten. Are people the better for it?

Scientific and technological advances have been so profound that if I treated a patient with an ulcer the way I did fifty years ago, the lawyers would soon be clambering over the transom—if there are any transoms left. But to understand the human spirit, doctors must look backward as well as forward, and looking backward offers a perspective of several thousand years of guidance.

Psychiatry reflects this division, too: manic-depressive illness, schizophrenia, and many other problems are surely neurobiological in origin and as deserving of medication and support as lupus or heart disease. Yet who can locate sorrow or joy or anxiety or ambition in the neurological impulses of the brain?

Where does empathy lie? Our contributors have generally avoided matters of faith as outside the purview of medicine; yet I read the same message in these essays: men and women are more than their bodies. Mind and spirit count in being human and in being sick. Social and economic forces may be as important to suffering as genes and trauma. To change the kinds of medical care doctors give, medical education must emphasize the social sciences and anthropology and sociology as much as physics and molecular biology, and the spiritual knowledge of philosophy and religion must be imparted, *before* medical school. We must give our students the broad education that will make them the kinds of physicians we all want.

Conclusion

Medical students now see little joy in medical practice and choose fields with sharply defined technical tasks where physicians act upon the patient as an object, not as *Thou*, but only as *It*. Few feel called upon to enter into the life of another person, to try to help.

Large changes are coming in the practice of medicine, and not all of the changes will be economic. Physicians' goals and attitudes must adapt to these changes if the joy of medicine is to be regained. So lost in work and duty—in office management even—physicians may have forgotten what attracted them to medicine—dare I say it?—the love of humanity and the hope of helping the suffering. But everyday work has destroyed empathy; the forms and the films, the techniques and the tasks, all the burdens of daily life in a complicated society dim that youthful vision. I hope that this book will encourage conversations about what physicians have lost by ignoring that which they cannot see. What some might call Spirit and others Grace may help to save doctors from cynicism.

The carpenter shapes the wood. Only a mystic would claim that the wood shapes the carpenter, although Michelangelo's unfinished statues in Florence suggest how the stone shapes the sculptor. But he was an artist, and physicians today are more like carpenters. The orthopedist who pauses in operating on a knee to marvel at how wondrously it is made may not get the job done. The surgeon who finds the universe in the patient's abdomen will turn away to write.

It need not be so. Medical practice may be splitting into two domains, that of caregivers and that of technicians. And some would ask whether medical training, now so long and arduous, is needed to remove a cataract or plumb the gut. Those who carry out procedures need no empathy, for it would only get in their way. For the rest, the doctors and nurses who care for—and sometimes cure—their fellow humans, the questions raised by this book remain to be answered.

Contributors

Joseph S. Alpert, M.D., received his B.A. from Yale University and his M.D. from Harvard Medical School. He trained in internal medicine and cardio-vascular disease at the Peter Bent Brigham Hospital in Boston and joined the staff there. Eventually, he served as the director of the Samuel A. Levine Cardiac Unit at that institution. In 1978, he was selected as the director of the division of cardiovascular medicine at the University of Massachusetts Medical School, where he was also the Edward Budnitz Professor of Cardiovascular Medicine. In 1992, he became the Robert S. and Irene P. Flinn Professor of Medicine and head of the department of medicine at the University of Arizona College of Medicine. Alpert has written widely on cardiovascular topics. For the last fifteen years, he has assisted his wife, Helle Mathiasen, in teaching a seminar for undergraduates entitled "Medicine and Literature: The Human Perspective."

George S. Bascom, M.D., recently retired from the practice of surgery after thirty-four years. His father was a doctor, as were three of his brothers and one of his sons. Preparation for a life in medicine included hoeing and haying for the college dairy during summers while in high school and later shingling, gandy dancing, carpentering, and playing football. In between, Bascom reluctantly attended school at Kansas State and Harvard Medical School and trained in surgery at Yale and elsewhere. His marriage and the arrival of five little boys complicated the poverty and obedience of internship and residency, and often moved his poor wife to wonder about life outside the nunnery.

The bitter breakup of a partnership, the death of a son, and the necessary losses of aging have been ameliorated by a wonderfully interesting life in surgery, the affection of his family, and warm friendships with classmates, colleagues, and patients.

Bascom has also found enormous satisfaction in writing poems, short stories, and essays. Though they please him and his uncritical friends, they have thus far eluded the glare of public attention outside Riley County, Kansas, and the barbs of the literati. Hope mingles with fear at the prospect of this brief emergence from total obscurity.

Rita Charon, M.D., is a general internist with an active inpatient and outpatient practice at Columbia-Presbyterian Medical Center in New York. Charon teaches medical students and residents medical interviewing skills and literature—both reading and writing—in attempts to bring them closer to the patients for whom they care. In addition to her clinical activities, Charon is a doctoral candidate in the department of English at Columbia University. She is writing a dissertation on the application of narrative frameworks to clinical practice. Her publications include linguistic studies of doctor-patient conversations, literary analyses of medical charts, and theoretical and practical aspects of teaching literature to doctors.

Mary Godenne McCrea Curnen, M.D., Dr.P.H., was born in Belgium and received her M.D. from Louvain University. She came to the United States in 1949 and pursued a career in virology at Yale University, working mainly with poliomyelitis and Coxsackie viruses. In 1973, after obtaining a Dr. of Public Health (epidemiology) from Columbia University, she devoted her research and teaching to cancer epidemiology. She returned to Yale in 1982 as director of the Connecticut Cancer Epidemiology Unit and medical director of the Connecticut Tumor Registry. She is presently clinical professor of epidemiology and pediatrics, continues her work in cancer epidemiology, and is assistant director of the Program for the Humanities in Medicine. Her publications have been in the fields of virology and cancer epidemiology.

Since 1985, she has been on the editorial board of the *Yale Journal of Biology and Medicine* and has served as guest editor of several special issues, including one devoted to the humanities in medicine. In 1990 she edited a book on her native country entitled *Modern Belgium*.

After the death of her first husband, John Falding McCrea, Ph.D., professor of microbiology at Yale University, she married Edward C. Curnen, Jr., M.D., Carpentier Professor of pediatrics emeritus, College of Physicians and Surgeons, Columbia University. Together they have seven children and ten grandchildren living in the United States and Australia.

Shimon M. Glick, M.D., is the father of six children and the grandfather of twenty. Glick is a native of New Jersey and a graduate of the Downstate Medical Center in Brooklyn. He trained in internal medicine at Maimonides Medical Center, Yale–New Haven Medical Center, and the Mount Sinai Hospital. He was subsequently a research fellow in endocrinology and nuclear medicine in the laboratory of Solomon Berson and Rosalyn Yalow (Nobel laureate) at the Bronx Veterans Administration Hospital. Before he immigrated to Israel in 1974, he was chief of endocrinology and then of medical services at the Coney Island Hospital in Brooklyn and clinical professor of medicine at the Downstate Medical Center. He was the founder and first president of the Society of Urban Physicians, a group of chiefs of service of New York City's municipal hospitals that organized to fight for improvements in patient care at those hospitals. In 1974, he became professor of medicine and chairman of the division of medicine at the newly founded Ben Gurion University Faculty of Health Sciences in Beer Sheva, Israel, where he was subsequently appointed dean. He currently heads the Center for Medical Education and a department of internal medicine at that school and teaches internal medicine, endocrinology, medical ethics, and communication skills.

Jodi Halpern, M.D., Ph.D., is a graduate of Yale College and the Yale University School of Medicine. She completed her psychiatry residency at the University of California, Los Angeles (UCLA), Neuropsychiatric Institute, and is a candidate for a doctorate in philosophy from Yale University. She integrates her interest in psychiatry and philosophy in her work on the physician-patient relationship. Halpern's doctoral thesis analyzes the ideal of "detached concern" in medicine. She argues that the ethical and cognitive aspects of medical practice require emotional engagement.

Currently, Halpern brings her theoretical background to empirical research on the impact of the changing structure of health services on medical ethics. She has also researched disruptions in communications in family therapy. Her interest in empathy is sustained by her clinical work, which is primarily psychodynamic in orientation.

Halpern leads weekly ethics rounds at the Neuropsychiatric Institute, teaches ethics at the UCLA Medical School, and serves on the ethics committee at the UCLA Medical Center.

Peter Kramer, M.D., is engaged in the private practice of outpatient psychiatry in Providence, Rhode Island. He is the author of *Listening to Prozac* (1993), a consideration of psychotherapeutic medication and its impact on the modern view of how people are constituted. His previous book is *Moments of Engagement: Intimate Psychotherapy in a Technological Age* (1989). Since 1985, Kramer has written a monthly column, "Practicing," for the *Psychiatric Times*. "Practicing" is the professional column most widely read by psychiatrists.

Kramer chairs the private practice committee of the American Psychiatric Association. He is associate clinical professor of psychiatry and human behavior at Brown University, where he teaches the basic course in individual psychotherapy for residents. He lectures widely on topics related to the mind-body interface in psychiatry.

Kramer graduated from Harvard College and then studied literature and philosophy at University College, London, on a Marshall Scholarship. After graduating from Harvard Medical School, he completed a medical internship at the University of Wisconsin and a psychiatry residency at Yale. Before joining the faculty at Brown University in 1982, he spent two-and-a-half years in public policy work, directing the division of science of the federal Alcohol, Drug Abuse, and Mental Health Administration.

Kramer is married to Rachel Schwartz, a public health researcher and policy analyst best known for her work in maternal and infant health. They have three children.

Michael A. LaCombe, M.D., was born in Ogdensburg, New York, in 1942. He graduated from the University of Rochester in 1964 and from the Harvard Medical School in 1968 and was chief resident in medicine at Strong Memorial Hospital in 1971–72. He has practiced general internal medicine full-time for twenty years, has lived in western Maine for eighteen years, and resides on a 450-acre farm with his wife, Ingrid, an orthopedic surgeon; their four children—Kristina, Mike, Thorsten, and David; and two Arabian horses, five dogs, two cats, a goat, and a pot-bellied pig named Cleopatra.

LaCombe has published more than seventy-five stories and essays in the *American Journal of Medicine* and the *Annals of Internal Medicine,* among other periodicals. He has also published one book and is associate editor of both the *American Journal of Medicine* and the *Annals.* He is a member of the board of directors of the American Board of Internal Medicine, where he serves on several committees, and he serves on two national committees for the American College of Physicians. With the Mayo Clinic, he has published one video of dramatic readings of his stories, and is at work on a second in collaboration with the American Board of Internal Medicine. Among other honors, he has been John S. Lawrence visiting professor at the University of California, Los Angeles, and Louis B. Matthews visiting professor at Dartmouth-Hitchcock Medical Center.

Richard L. Landau, M.D., Ph.D., was born on August 8, 1916. He received his B.S. and M.D. degrees from Washington University in St. Louis in 1940. He completed his internship, one year of residency in medicine, and a one-year fellowship in endocrinology working with Allan Kenyon at the University of Chicago Clinics in 1943. Following three years in the 40th Infantry Division, he returned to the department of medicine at the University of Chicago, where he has remained. He became an emeritus professor in 1987, but continues to practice and teach medicine and endocrinology.

Landau's research was concentrated on the analysis of urinary steroids, the metabolic influence of androgens, estrogen, and progesterone, the physiology of pregnancy, and other aspects of reproductive physiology in humans.

For more than twenty years he served as director of the clinical research center (starting prior to funding by the National Institutes of Health), and he was the chairman of the institutional review board responsible for overseeing clinical research for the first fifteen years of its existence.

In 1973 he joined his wife, Claire, who was managing editor of *Perspectives in Biology and Medicine*, as editor and remains active in that position.

Jeanne LeVasseur, R.N., M.S.N., F.N.P., is a family nurse practitioner and assistant clinical professor at Yale University School of Nursing. She holds an M.F.A. in writing and uses poetry and fiction to teach nursing students about the experience of illness.

Joanne Lynn, M.D., M.A., recently joined Dartmouth-Hitchcock Medical Center as a professor of medicine and of community and family medicine, a senior associate in the Center for the Evaluative Clinical Sciences, and associate director of the Center for the Aging. She was previously a hospice and long-term care physician while director of the Center for Aging Studies and Services at George Washington University. She is co-director of SUPPORT, the Study to Understand Prognosis and Performances for Outcomes and Risks of Treatments, and was assistant director of the Presidents's Commission for the Study of Ethical Problems in Medicine and Biomedical and Behavioral Research.

Helle Mathiasen, Ph.D., was born in Copenhagen, Denmark. She was awarded the Cand.Mag. degree (more than an M.A. but less than a Ph.D.) in English and Greek from Copenhagen University in 1967. After emigrating from Denmark to the United States, she studied Colonial American literature and society at Tufts University, obtaining her Ph.D. in English from Tufts in 1974. She has lectured on, written about, and taught English, American literature, Scandinavian literature, and philosophy, most recently for fourteen years in the Boston College Honors Program. Since 1978, she and her husband, Joseph S. Alpert, M.D., have taught a course together and lectured together on topics in the medical humanities. She is presently teaching in the humanities program at the University of Arizona, Tucson.

Harold J. Morowitz, Ph.D., is Robinson Professor of biology and natural philosophy at George Mason University. He received his Ph.D. from Yale University and was a member of the Yale faculty from 1955 to 1987. His research deals with the thermodynamic basis of biology and the origin of life. Morowitz writes a monthly column for *Hospital Practice*. His recent books are *Facts of Life: Science and the Abortion Controversy* (with James Trefil, 1992), *The Beginnings of Cellular Life* (1992), and *Entropy and the Magic Flute* (1993).

Enid Peschel, Ph.D., is assistant professor (adjunct) of internal medicine and co-director of the Program for Humanities in Medicine at Yale University School of Medicine. She received her B.A. from Brown University and her Ph.D. from Harvard University. She is co-editor, with Richard E. Peschel, Carol W. Howe, and James W. Howe of *Neurobiological Disorders in Children and Adolescents* (1992). In November 1992, she coordinated the Yale–National Institutes of Mental Health Continuing Medical Education conference entitled "Recent Findings from the Neuroscience Revolution: Implications for Autism, Schizophrenia, Affective Disorders, and More in Children and Young Adults." She is currently the course coordinator for the Yale Continuing Medical Education Conference on a similar topic. She is co-author, with her husband, Richard E. Peschel, of *When a Doctor Hates a Patient and Other Chapters in a Young Physician's Life* (1986). Among her ten books and edited and translated volumes are *Medicine and Literature* (1980), Arthur Rimbaud's *A Season in Hell: The Illuminations* (1973), *Four French Symbolist Poets: Baudelaire, Rimbaud, Verlaine, Mallarmé* (1981), and "A Selection from the Program for Humanities in Medicine, Yale University School of Medicine," a volume of the *Yale Journal of Biology and Medicine* (1992).

Richard E. Peschel, M.D., Ph.D., is professor of therapeutic radiology at Yale University School of Medicine. Peschel received his M.D. from Yale University School of Medicine and his Ph.D. in nuclear physics from Yale University. He has published more than 120 articles, chapters, and books on medicine, nuclear physics, literature and medicine, opera and medicine, and neurobiological disorders. He is a co-editor of *Neurobiological Disorders in Children and Adolescents* (1992). He is also the co-author, with Enid Peschel, of *When a Doctor Hates a Patient and Other Chapters in a Young Physician's Life* (1986). In 1988, he received a Deems Taylor Award from the American Society of Composers, Authors, and Publishers (ASCAP) for an article he wrote with Enid Peschel, "The Castrati in Opera," published in the *Opera Quarterly* (1987). Peschel is currently a co-editor of *The Urologic Cancer Textbook* (In press).

Stanley Joel Reiser, M.D., M.P.A., Ph.D., is the Griff T. Ross Professor of humanities and technology in health care at the University of Texas Health Science Center at Houston. He received his A.B. degree from Columbia University, his M.D. from the State University of New York and Downstate Medical Center, his M.P.A. from the Kennedy School of Government, Harvard University, and his Ph.D. in the history of science from Harvard University.

His first academic post was on the faculty of Harvard University, holding appointments at the Medical School and College, and also at Massachusetts General Hospital. His teaching and research centered on the humanistic, technological, and policy dimensions of health care. In 1982, Reiser left his post as associate professor at Harvard to move to Houston, as professor and director of the Program on Humanities and Technology in Health Care. His publications, as author or co-editor, include the books *Medicine and the Reign of Technology* (1978); *Ethics in Medicine* (1977); *The Machine at the Bedside* (1984); *Integrity in Health Care Institutions* (1990); and *The Ethical Dimensions of the Biological Sciences* (1993). He is currently the co-editor of the *International Journal of Technology Assessment in Health Care.*

Deborah St. James, B.A., is medical editor at Miles Editorial Services. She attended Cornell University and holds a B.A. in English from the University of Akron. Deborah is a writer, editor, and educator. She has taught English, English as a second language, and technical writing, and she was senior editor of *Better Health* magazine. She currently teaches writing and speaking skills to physicians and other health care personnel. She is the author of *Writing and Speaking for Excellence: A Practical Guide for Physicians.*

Howard M. Spiro, M.D., was born in Cambridge, Massachusetts, in 1924. He graduated from Harvard College and Harvard Medical School and received his postgraduate training at the Peter Bent Brigham Hospital and at Massachusetts General Hospital before moving to New Haven, Connecticut, in 1955. An academic clinical gastroenterologist, Spiro established the Section of Gastroenterology at the Yale University School of Medicine in 1955 and headed this section until 1982. In 1982, he became director of the Program for Humanities in Medicine. Spiro is probably best known for his textbook, *Clinical Gastroenterology* (4th ed., 1993), but he has also authored *Doctors, Patients, and Placebos* (1986) and, with Harvey Mandell, *When Doctors Get Sick* (1987). He is proud of the fact that two of his four children are practicing psychiatrists and that one is a nurse-practitioner. His wife, Marian, who has kept him from too great a degree of pomposity, retired after twenty years as a schoolteacher and is now a carpenter.

John Stone, M.D., was born in Jackson, Mississippi. He received his B.A. from Millsaps College and his M.D. from Washington University School of Medicine. He did his postgraduate training at the University of Rochester and at Emory University. Since 1969, Stone has taught at Emory University School of Medicine, where he is now professor of medicine (cardiology) and associate dean. He has also served as visiting lecturer for the English department at Emory. He has spoken and read from his work in all parts of the country.

Stone's poetry is collected in three books: *The Smell of Matches* (1972), *In All*

This Rain (1980), and *Renaming the Streets* (1985). A book of his essays, *In The Country of Hearts*, was published in 1990. Stone's poems have been published widely and also anthologized. His essays have appeared nationally in such publications as the *New York Times Magazine, Discover,* and *MD* magazine.

Stone served as co-editor (with Richard Reynolds) for an anthology of literature and medicine called *On Doctoring: Stories, Poems, Essays* (1991). The volume is presented annually as a gift from the Robert Wood Johnson Foundation to every first-year medical student in the United States.

David R. Vance, M.A., is a lecturer in philosophy at Central Connecticut State University. He holds an M.A. in philosophy from the University of Washington and is a Ph.D. candidate at the University of Connecticut. His research interests are in the application of hermeneutical conceptions of understanding to questions of social ethics.

Index